In *Richard Simmons' Never-Say-Diet Cookbook* you'll get:

• More information on food and cooking techniques . . . lists of foods to indulge in and those to avoid . . . guidelines on portions

• Over one hundred new and exciting recipes that follow Richard's formula to weight success . . . recipes never before in print or on TV . . . easy-to-make, great-tasting dishes from Richard's own file and from those of fellow "live-it" weight-fighters, to slim your figure and please your family... all pre-tested and pre-tasted in the author's taste kitchen

• Tongue-in-cheek quizzes that will make you laugh off pounds and probe your attitudes toward food and mealtimes

• Eating tips for both house folk and office workers . . . ways to solve coffee-break cravings and four-o'clock munchies . . . solutions to common lunchtime problems . . . helpful advice for getting kids and other family members to eat right.

You'll find photo-illustrated exercises to change your life-style, along with inspiring testimonials from former weight-fighters now on their way to slimness. There's a soap opera script to challenge the networks and a dozen luncheon recipes to go with it ("Guiding Bite," "One Loaf to Live," plus others).

You'll learn how to change your food habits, your life-style, and your figure; but, most of all, you'll learn to create healthful, weight-conscious, and delicious meals.

Richard Simmons'

Never-Say-Diet Cookbook

WARNER BOOKS

A Warner Communications Company

Dedication

I'd like to dedicate this book to my parents and my brother Lenny, even though he's still perfect. My mom is seventy-one years old and my dad is eighty-five and never once did they consider putting me in a home or giving me away to fat gypsies. I love you.

Copyright © 1982 by Richard Simmons, Inc.
All rights reserved.
Warner Books, Inc., 666 Fifth Avenue, New York, NY 10103

W A Warner Communications Company

Printed in the United States of America
First trade paperback printing: May 1983
10 9 8 7 6 5 4 3 2 1

Library of Congress Cataloging in Publication Data

Simmons, Richard.
  Richard Simmons' Never-say-diet cookbook.

  1. Reducing diets—Recipes.   2. Reducing exercises.
3. Reducing—Psychological aspects.   I. Title.
II. Title: Never-say-diet cookbook.
RM222.2.S546   1982   641.5'635   81-19640
ISBN 0-446-37078-9 (USA)   AACR2
ISBN 0-446-37553-5 (Canada)

Book design by H. Roberts Design
Illustrations on pages 94, 96, 200, 202 and 206 by Howard Roberts

Acknowledgments

Acknowledgments are really hard to write. You stay up half the night trying to remember if you forgot anyone, terrified of leaving out the name of someone really important to you. Like your third grade teacher who taught you how to type. Or the English teacher who gave me a D. Then you stay up more nights worring that no one is going to read the acknowledgments. Do you know anyone who reads acknowledgments?

I happen to be one of the few people who do read acknowledgments. And I have a personal gripe about them. Authors thank people like Erma Klotzman, but they never tell you who Erma is to them and what she did to earn the author's thanks. So you get bored and end up staying up even more nights fantasizing about Erma Klotzman. Is she young, is she old? Does she have blond frizzy hair and glasses? I mean, who is she?

So here is my personal list of acknowledgments. If I've left anyone out, I've provided a space at the end of the list for corrections. I really didn't do everything in this book all by myself so there are several people I'd like to thank. And you better read every name because there just might be a quiz in the book about them later on. In alphabetical order, I'd like to thank:

*Barbara Bartman, my personal friend, and Auntie Barbara, who has believed in me from the beginning and has always been there for me.

*Woody and Nora Fraser, the producers of *The Richard Simmons Show*, the "married team" who actually went out and bought—retail no less—eighty-seven copies of my last book to give as Christmas presents to their friends. And they are my bestest friends.

*Peggy Ganz, my girl Friday, Saturday, and Sunday, who does everything and gets paid like a vice-president.

*Suzy Kalter, my collaborator, who helps my words come out right. (She won every spelling bee from kindergarten through high school.)

*Howard Kaminsky, Mark Greenberg, and Jonathon Lazear, who promised me, if this book did as well as *Never-Say-Diet,* I could use the lobby of the Warner Communications building as an exercise studio for New Yorkers.

*Allen Lenard and Bruce Littel, my attorney and my accountant, without whom life would be more difficult.

*Elyse Lewin and Robert Blakeman, who photographed this book and made sure none of my pimples showed.

*Nansey Neiman, my editor at Warner Books, who lost seventeen pounds while working on this book.

*Anita Nuñez, my home economist, who cooks on the show and who made every recipe in this book and tasted them. And didn't gain any weight doing it!

*Edie Rome, Arnold Lipsman, Rebecca Segal, and Doreen Lauer for making sure people know who I am. (Except I'll never forgive them for setting me up as the centerfold in *Field & Stream.*)

*Nancy Simmons, my costume mistress (no, she's not my wife), who takes my fantasies and turns them into real characters on my show and on these pages.

* _____ Fill in your name or the name of anyone you think I may have left out, because I couldn't have done it without you!

Contents

WARNING

Please do not add any additional ingredients (fattening or foreign) to any of the Live-It recipes in this cookbook. Never-Say-Diet agents will be making house-to-house inspections, and if chocolate sprinkles, powdered sugar, or greasy spots are found smearing the pages, you will be in big trouble. You will be automatically put on probation, your book will be confiscated, an unpleasant announcement will be made in your neighborhood telling all who can hear that you are not staying on your weight-loss program, and you will be mortally embarrassed. And I don't think either of us wants that to happen.

Live-It *(liv-it)* Expression invented by Richard Simmons meant to replace the word diet *(dī-et)*. The Live-It is an ongoing, not temporary, food and exercise program that combines a volume food plan with a rigorous exercise program. What you eat, when you eat, and how much you exercise can control weight, says Simmons, so there is no need to count calories, figure out carbs, or match up enzymes. You can Live-It—and love it.

Start Here

I read my first cookbook when I was three years old. Okay, I couldn't really read at that age, but I memorized and acted out reading while I turned the pages. This is very common for children of three—they memorize Dr. Seuss. I am Sam. Sam I am. Do you like green eggs and ham? Well, I liked green eggs and ham, so I memorized a cookbook. Dr. Seuss was fine for other people, but I was much more interested in this red and white gingham notebook with the shiny color pictures called *The Better Homes & Gardens Cookbook*. It was my mother's, and it was not only a kitchen companion but my best friend.

Other kids went on to *Peter Pan*, Dick and Jane, and *The Catcher in the Rye*. I just kept on poring over the pictures in the cookbook. I would spend all my after-school time drooling over the pictures of the Martha Washington cake or the macaroni and cheese casserole with bacon bits and pimiento. While the other kids were having trouble with hard words like *haven't*, *umbrella*, and *neighborhood*, I was struggling over the correct pronunciation of *soufflé*, *sauté*, and *marinate*. I promise you, I was the only kid in the first grade whose flash cards were made on recipe cards that had the words FROM THE KITCHEN OF MILTON T. SIMMONS.

I actually got my own very first cookbook when I was about twelve. We were at a garage sale, and my mom was looking at this crazy collection of bottles that had been turned into lamps and my father was thumbing through the jazz albums (two for a quarter) and I discovered the rows and rows of books. Mom thought I was looking for *The Adventures of Tom Sawyer,* but when I came upon Peg Bracken's *I Hate to Cook Book,* I fell in love.

By the time I was fourteen, I had a complete set of cookbooks. You have to remember that this was in the early sixties and the cookbook revolution was just beginning. The old-fashioned cookbooks had these funny little line drawings in them of things like a measuring cup, a whisk, and two eggs, as if they were a still life by Cézanne. But my mother had come to realize that the only way she could get me to sit down with a good book was to buy me a good cookbook (with color pictures, please). So she did the buying for about a year. Then suddenly it got to be Mother's Day, and I was old enough to go shopping for her on my own. I wandered all through this big department store in New Orleans: I considered stationery; I considered perfume; maybe a nightie with maribou feathers? Then I had the most brilliant idea of my entire fifteen years. I would buy her a cookbook! (One I didn't have.) As fast as my chubby thighs would carry me I dashed down three flights of moving es-

calator stairs to the basement book department, conveniently located next to the housewares department. As I approached the book department I realized that something very special was happening. There was an in-store demonstration. Only I didn't know that that's what they called them then. All I knew was, there was a huge crowd of people all gathered around a table, and standing there—behind a red tablecloth and an aluminum wok—was Madame Ku. Madame Ku was the proprietress of a local Chinese bistro, and she had been brought in by the store during United Nations Week to teach Chinese cooking and promote a little cookbook that included recipes from around the world.

I had never seen a cooking demonstration before (outside of my home, that is) and I was immediately enthralled. Madame Ku had the dexterity of a snake charmer. She danced that little cleaver around the chopping board, she did kung fu on some water chestnuts, and she stir-fried a few morsels that were soon passed around to the crowd. I suddenly realized why cooking demonstrations were so popular. You got to have a free lunch!

Madame Ku changed my life. There she was talking up a storm, waving that cleaver wildly, passing around the best dumplings, which she called *dim sum,* and selling a zillion books. Not only did I buy a book, but I got a wok, and a set of chopsticks for each member of the family. (Actually I got three sets; I thought Lenny could eat with his hands—it would serve him right for being so perfect.) I bought a cleaver and had my initials engraved on the handle and went home immediately to present my gift and start fixing Chinese food for my friends and family.

Ever since that long-ago day, I have been a sucker for cooking demonstrations. I can stand there for a full half hour, biting my knuckles, waiting for them to pass the samples around. I've even developed my own special technique of crowd rotation so I can be the first person they pass the tray to. And I'm not cheap about it. I always buy the cookbook after I've had the free eats.

To this day I'm the same way. I will buy a cookbook if it:

a. is advertised on television.

b. has beautiful color pictures.

c. is sold in conjunction with a cooking demonstration.

d. is on display at the checkout counter in my grocery store.

e. is mentioned by some celebrity on a talk show.

f. sounds like something I've never heard of before.

g. offers great low-calorie gourmet meals.

h. is devoted to some country or region that sounds exotic.

Need I go on? Do I need to tell you that some people have rooms in their homes they call Libraries because they are too embarassed to call them Cookbook Rooms. They are lined with wooden shelves that I promise you are solely devoted to cookbooks. They cannot count how many cookbooks they own. They rarely use them. Sometimes if they can't sleep at night, they take a few down from the shelves and fondle them lovingly—the books are old friends and can give a great feeling of security. They have probably tried at least one—but not more than five—recipes from each of these books. But mostly they buy books for sensual gratification.

I have the problem myself. My own Library is in my kitchen. When I make a recipe from a book, I invariably fall into what I call the Cookbook Crisis. I hold in my hands the world's most beautiful cookbook. I open to the page of the recipe of my choice. I stare at the photograph for thirty-five minutes, getting close enough to the page to smell the finished product. Then I follow the directions carefully, step by step, never taking shortcuts. In the end I sit on my kitchen stool and stare at my creation. My eyes roll from my dish to the picture to the back of my head and back again. I blink. Maybe I'm tired. I look at my dish, the picture, and then my dish again. Where did I go wrong? How could I be so stupid? Why does my plate look so different from the one in the picture?

But I'm not a quitter. So I throw out my meager attempt at following directions and I start over. Once again I stare from my plate to the picture and back again. Still not right. How could I have done it wrong again? I dig through the trash and resurrect the mess I threw away an hour before. I compare the two failures. They are similar. But they look nothing like the photograph. I am a failure.

So I go out and buy another cookbook with the hope that this time, maybe this time, I can come up with something as glorious as the picture that inspired me.

I will always buy cookbooks that promise:
• that the recipes are easy.
• that the recipes are quick.
• that I, too, no matter how limited my abilities, can accomplish the recipes.
• that any child above the age of six can make the recipes with stunning results.

This process went on for many, many years. I became a cookbooksomaniac. (That's a lot like a nymphomaniac—I can't get no satisfaction.) I went through many years of my adult life like this—feeling inadequate, thinking I had a serious problem I couldn't tell anyone about. I even considered going into psychoanalysis to see if I had a more serious problem related to my feelings about my mother. Then a friend of mine in the cookbook publishing business told me about the Cookbook Conspiracy.

I am about to save you the years of agony I have endured. Here and now I will tell you what I learned. So hold your breath—you will barely believe this.

It seems that food is the most difficult thing in the world to photograph. More difficult than beautiful women, babies, or animals. The ingredients melt under the lights. The pouf goes woof in a matter of seconds. The gravy stops oozing and starts to gurgle. The crystallized sugar begins to sweat and get wet and lumpy. The food has no sparkle and no pizzazz. Even photographed in black and white it has no oomph. If you printed pictures of food the way it really photographs, no one would ever buy a cookbook or a magazine again. In fact, few people would ever eat again.

Obviously this is no way to run a food business, so the cookbook publishers and magazine editors of the food world united and began to cheat on the preparation of the food so it would photograph better.

You've heard about Lauren Hutton and that little piece of plastic she puts in the gap between her two front teeth when she's being photographed, so no one knows about the imperfection in her ivories. Well, food editors began to cheat with food. It was all harmless. They just started using shaving cream instead of whipped cream. (Shaving cream has a lot more body, and it holds up better under the lights. It looks really yummy too.) They started dipping fruits and vegetables in vegetable oil or baby oil so they'd sparkle as we imagine they did while still attached to the tree or the stalk where they came from. They used marking pens to color up so-so looking foods or they went entirely to plaster of Paris so they wouldn't have to bother with the real thing at all. Have you ever been to a bakery and taken a good hard stare at that scrumptious five-tier wedding cake they have on display? The one that congratulates Jane and Jimmy, with the tiny little bride and groom statuette on the top and the butter-cream roses? Well, guess what, folks—that's a fake cake.

But it sells cakes. And the food tricks sell the books and the magazines they are supposed to sell. And the only time it hurts is when you stand at home, making recipe after recipe, getting more and more frustrated because you can't duplicate the picture.

I'd like to think I have a little more integrity than all that. It's hard enough to make really good-looking, good-tasting, low-calorie food. To deceive people into thinking it looks like something it doesn't is an insult to everyone. So here we are: you and I. The cookbook you have in your hands, the *Never-Say-Diet Cookbook*, does not have one touched-up photograph in it. There will be very few food pictures in the book, and what you see is what you get. None of these pictures has been tampered with by man or beast. Each photograph was taken as the food came out of the oven or off the counter. We might have let it cool (steam does fog up the camera lens) but we did nothing else to it.

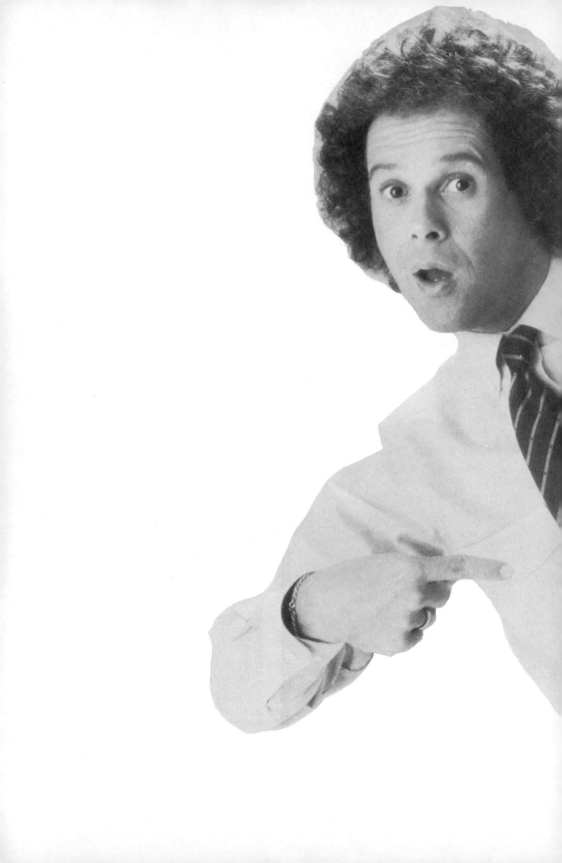

Meet Your
Live-It Life

TRUE CONFESSIONS

Okay, everybody, let's talk about it. Let's get it out in the open right now and do some serious one-on-one communicating. You're thinking it and I *know* you're thinking it, so we better sit right down and talk about it. No need to sit right down and write yourself a letter. We're going to come clean. I happen to think these things are really important and have to be brought out in the open, discussed eye to eye, man to man, and appetizer to appetizer.

You bought this book because you read the first one. Or someone told you to buy this new book because they liked the old one.

You plunked down your hard-earned sixteen bucks and now you're worried. You know that the sequel to a great movie is never as good as the first movie. You know why that sequel to *Gone With the Wind* (there really is one, you know) was never filmed. You know that *Son of Frankenstein* wasn't anything compared to *Frankenstein*. And now you're worried that this book isn't going to be as good as *Never-Say-Diet*. You're afraid that you've wasted your money and that you're going to be sorry. You will try to compare this book to the first book, you will try to measure me by my (and your) previous success. You will never even consider that this book isn't *The Godfather, Part III.*

So stop right here. There's something I better tell you.

Relax.

You're going to like this book. (I hope you love it.)

But more importantly, this book is not a sequel. It's a partner. It's an addition to *Never-Say-Diet.* Together they are one. Sort of like Abbott and Costello or Adam and Eve. They go together like peanut butter and jelly—oops, sorry about that.

And besides, I'm not running a competition here. So it's not even a case of one book being better than the other. Each book is different. This book, the *Never-Say-Diet Cookbook,* is an extension of the same thinking, but it is not out to outdo any other book.

Never-Say-Diet explained my way of combining exercise, mental attitude, and a sensible food plan to bring you a weight loss and a new life-style. This new book, the *Never-Say-Diet Cookbook,* will give you more information about food and cooking techniques and will supplement your daily existence on the Live-It of your choice by introducing 101 new and approved recipes for losing weight.

These are not recipes you've seen on television, by the way. (My show or anybody else's.) These are brand-new, exclusive recipes, created solely for you and this book. Many of them are my recipes. (And not my mother's, so don't you believe her.) Many of the recipes come from friends of mine who have lost weight on the Live-It and have been kind enough to share their recipes with all of us. (Bless their hearts.)

When I first sat down to plan this book, I originally thought to have a big fancy contest, asking people to send me their Live-It recipes. It would be a lot like the search for the actress to play Scarlett O'Hara or the hunt for a new face for Annie. Millions of Americans would respond to my plea for creative recipes that were fun, easy to make, nutritious, inexpensive, and made with low-calorie foods as outlined in my Live-It plan. I was going to get foods that tasted good, that everyone would enjoy, and that would make my book a necessity in every cook's kitchen. I wasn't dreaming of recipes for shredded carrots, water-packed tuna salad, or green peas with parsley. I wanted good—even gourmet—recipes that would be a joy to all who tasted them.

So I put out a few feelers. I quietly asked around town for recipes. I even offered money for these recipes. I mean, you can't do any better than that, can you?

Well, yes you can. While I thought this was going to be as easy as pie (excuse the expression), the people who were sending in recipes ended up pleading no contest. After three weeks of nonstop reading, I realized I had enough material to write a book on zoos of the world. No one, I mean, no one, sent me a recipe I would serve to myself, my dog (if I had one), or guests in my home.

I don't want to hurt anyone's feelings, but those recipes were real bad. I mean, real bad. Not good at all.

You don't believe me?

Okay, try this one. And this is a real honest-to-goodness entry.

Cottage Cheese Delight

1 pound cottage cheese
1 4-ounce box Jell-O (any flavor; my
    favorite is raspberry)
1 12-ounce can crushed pineapple
1 9-ounce container Cool Whip
2 8-ounce cups Kraft miniature
    marshmallows (optional)

1. Make Jell-O according to directions
   on box.
2. Add cottage cheese.
3. Stir in Cool Whip and
   crushed pineapple.
4. For extra flavor, add marshmallows (I
   do!).
5. Chill and serve.

Serves: One

I swear to you, this is a real recipe that someone sent to me. (I even had to get a lawyer's approval to reprint it here.) I mean, can you believe this was someone's idea of a recipe to lose weight on? Did you get a look at the proportions? This isn't meant to be a snack for thirty-four starving third-graders. This is for one person. One very large, unhappy person.

After looking at that recipe and hundreds like it, I began to understand why people take a package out of the freezer or open a can or drop something into boiling water and think they're going to eat a good meal.

No one has ever come up with great-tasting, easy-to-make, non-fattening foods before.

And let me tell you, this was a terrible thing to realize. In fact, the realization nearly broke my heart. I felt I had failed. At first, I must admit, I thought the recipes I stumbled upon were jokes—you know, a few wild cards sent in by one clown or another. But as they piled up on my navy blue living room carpet, I dismally realized I would have been lucky to have been plagued by jokers. I fell deeper and deeper into depression. And I'm not easily depressed.

It just killed me to think no one was paying attention to me, hearing my plea to eat sensibly. Down in my heart I feel that if I fail, then you fail; and if you fail, it makes me an even bigger failure. And let me tell you, that's a pretty heavy load—not at all good for the self-esteem. Me claiming to be the Weight Saint and all that. If people are really cooking meals like Cottage Cheese Delight, then I must be doing something wrong.

Except that I did lose weight myself. And I know lots of other people have lost weight and kept it off. So rather than jump off some bridge over troubled water, I began to go through my mail. I put together names, addresses, and phone numbers of people who had lost weight. I contacted people who had lost one hundred pounds. I spoke to people who had lost thirty pounds. And people who lost somewhere in between. I spoke to the kind of losers I call winners. And I asked them to send me their recipes.

And then it began to work. No more Cottage Cheese Delight. I started getting some great recipes. The kind you'll find in this book. And I've included them along with my personal recipes to make this a testimonial cookbook.

The recipes in this book were tested three times in an antiseptic test kitchen, just the way they should have been. But long before they ever got to the testing grounds, they were tested at home and at table by real people. What you have, collected in this book, are the recipes I personally use to maintain my weight and the recipes of people from all over this country who have lost weight cooking these meals. And you can't ask for a better recommendation than that, now, can you, Julia?

But just to make sure you're ready to start cooking the Richard Simmons way, I want to see if you're attuned to the Live-It. If you pass this quiz, congratulations, I am really proud. You thumb on right through to the next section. But if you flunk, well, guys, there's only one thing you can do: Study *Never-Say-Diet* every night for one week. Then requiz yourself. When you pass, proceed to the next section.

Okay? Ready? Pen out? No, don't use that pencil. You might cheat and erase. All right, here goes.

1. **A Live-It is:**
a. a typographical error referring to a hippie love-in.
b. a new type of food plan that ends dieting.
c. a housekeeper who sleeps in your home.

2. **Americans are all overweight because they:**
a. inherited a lot of fat cells from the Pilgrims.
b. eat the wrong foods at the wrong time of day.
c. can't stop themselves from eating apple pie.

3. **The girl I really wanted to date was:**
a. Susan Karp.
b. Juanita Wasserman.
c. Gloria Verstein.

4. **For breakfast each morning you eat:**
a. four blueberry pancakes, two fried eggs (over easy), three strips of bacon, a large glass of orange juice, and two cups of coffee—with cream and sugar, please.
b. one scrambled egg, a slice of toast, fresh juice.
c. I never eat breakfast; I'm on a diet.

5. **You believe in beginning each day with:**
a. *Captain Kangaroo.*
b. a smile, some stretches, and a good breakfast.
c. a box of sugar-coated cereal and a few phone calls while watching a morning news-program.

6. **Lenny is:**
a. my parakeet.
b. my brother.
c. a movie starring Valerie Perrine.

7. **Every day at midmorning you:**
a. turn on the soaps, grab some Pepperidge Farm (real pudding!) cake from the fridge, and get comfortable.
b. watch *The Richard Simmons Show.*
c. begin to think about lunch.

8. You think a Mini Pushup is:
a. a frozen yogurt on a stick.
b. an exercise to perform religiously.
c. a short skirt worn in England in 1965, when mod was "in."

9. At lunch you like to:
a. eat a big fancy meal, preferably French.
b. eat a well-balanced meal you can work off later.
c. grab some leftovers from the fridge so you can make a hasty return to the television set or the book you are presently reading.

10. After lunch the best thing to do is:
a. get right back to office or housework.
b. plan an activity that will burn off calories.
c. have some dessert and take a nice nap.

11. You think that exercise programs:
a. are good for people who want to develop muscles.
b. are the key to your good health and trim figure.
c. are too expensive because you never go anyway.

12. My hometown is:
a. New Mexico.
b. New Orleans.
c. New York.

13. You think Yo-Yo Syndrome is:
a. a new Olympic event.
b. a deadly habit of gaining and losing weight.
c. a child's habit of popping up and down out of bed when he doesn't want to go to sleep at night.

14. When you go to a restaurant for dinner:
a. you make your choice based on who's paying.
b. you stick to your food plan.
c. you order a lot of everything because the food is better than what you make at home.

15. Each night before you go to sleep, you:
a. have a glass of warm milk.
b. do some stretching exercises and say your prayers.
c. have a little snack and smoke a cigarette.

WARNING: Some of the answers to this test may look like they are obvious and I am a dodo for asking. But the answers you should pick are the ones that are true for you, not the ones that you think will improve your score. Got it? Now go back and change the ones where you picked what you thought was a good answer even if it wasn't true. Thank you. Now, don't you feel better about that?

Okay. To score, give yourself ten (10) points for each (a) answer, five (5) points for each (b) answer, and twenty (20) points for each (c) answer.

If your score is 75–90 points

Good for you. You go to the head of the class. You must have memorized *Never-Say-Diet* and really done your homework. I am truly proud. You understand the Live-It and you're ready for this book immediately. God bless you.

If your score is 95–125 points

Not bad, not bad at all. You could use a bit of a brushup, but I think you're running with me. Take a quick glance at the exercise pages of *Never-Say-Diet* and brush up on the section on food plans.

If your score is 130–165

I beg your pardon. I don't know how to break this to you nicely, but you seem to have a few bad habits (or a good bit of misinformation) locked into your brain that are keeping you from being as slim as you can be. You better read *Never-Say-Diet* (it's in paperback!) and requiz yourself. Get that score down a bit, please.

If your score is 170–250 points

All right, smarty pants, I've got your number. You're the one who walks through a bookstore, looks at all the diet books, leafs through the pages, and then puts the books down again with your chocolate pudding thumbprints on them. You shrug your hefty shoulders and say diet books don't work and are a waste of money. You've never even read *Never-Say-Diet* and you've all but given up on yourself and your future. If you buy this book, you may make one recipe, but then you'll put the book on the shelf with your

418 other cookbooks and never use it again. So don't waste your money. You won't be ready to really take advantage of the good things in this book until you get your mental attitude in better shape. Start with *Never-Say-Diet* before you buy this book. You can get control of your figure if you're willing to work at it, so give me a chance, huh?

If your score is 255 or over

Waddle, do not walk, to your nearest airline and buy yourself a one-way ticket to Beverly Hills. Meet me at the Anatomy Asylum, and let's get to work on you immediately. You've got a long way to go baby, but I'm going to help you.

SAY HELLO TO THE LIVE-IT

It's the word *diet* I hate so much. How can you be fond of anything with the word *die* in it? And I've been through so much on the seven zillion diets I personally tried and tested that I really did almost die. So you and I are making a pact to eradicate the word *diet* from the vocabulary of the world.

Our substitute? *Live-It*, of course.

The Live-It is my answer to the diet. It's a lifelong sensible plan. It doesn't mean you're just "on" the Live-It and then you go back to "normal," whatever that is. That, in essence, is what's wrong with diets in the first place.

The Live-It is an entire way of life: It's a volume food plan, an exercise plan, and a whole mental attitude. When you know you can take off weight and keep it off, you have a determination that will make you triumphant. That's what the Live-It is all about.

So let's take a look at the various parts of the Live-It that you're going to need to focus on while making the transition from grievous sinner (dieter) to thin and healthy. Come with me, I've got a few friends to introduce you to. They're going to change your life. And you'll be a lot happier person. I promise.

MEET YOUR LIVE-IT FOODS

Because the Live-It is not a diet, there's no such thing as calorie counting, good and bad carbohydrates, in foods or out foods, or good foods or bad foods. On the Live-It, you can pretty much eat anything you want to eat—you just have to be careful of how much of it you eat, when you eat it, and how much exercise you do before and after eating it.

But there are certain foods that are better for you than others. So I want you to meet them, say hello, get to know their relatives, and ask them to join you and your family at mealtime.

Shake Hands with Mr. and Mrs. Chicken: I sure hope you like chicken, because chicken likes you. And so do the relatives turkey and game hen. There are a few, uh, black sheep in the family you ought to ignore—duck and goose—but on the whole, the chickens are a very nice flock of friends. Chicken provides protein, A and B vitamins, iron and calcium and, more importantly, it's low in saturated fat. Don't forget to take the skin off your little chickie bird after it's been cooked but before it's on your fork.

Be a Live-It Liver Lover: Don't tell me how prejudiced you are about liver. Well, *ugh* to you too. Liver happens to be one of the best friends your body will ever have. And, as we all know, you've got a liver of your own. But I suggest you get well-acquainted with someone else's liver—preferably a chicken's rather than a calf's. Liver is a real beauty-and-health food—it's rich in vitamins, proteins, has the good things that make your nails grow, your skin glow, your hair shine and, on top of all that, it's filled with iron. And we all know that while ironing may not be good for our health (boring, huh?) iron is what makes your body hum. Women often have a deficiency of iron to begin with. So take a look at some of our tasty liver treats later on in the book and give your body a treat. Liver once a week won't kill you.

Meet the Meats: It's a well known fact that red meat just isn't as good for you as chicken and fish. In fact, Americans eat far too much red meat and could all stand to cut back on the steaks and hamburgers (and the fries and the ketchup and the . . .). It's hard, I know that. There are some people who consider themselves the meat-and-potatoes type who can't even stand the thought of a day without meat, let alone a life without meat. I'm not about to tell you to become a vegetarian or to give up burgers. But I am reminding you of what you already know: Too much red meat is dangerous for you. So follow these tips when picking a Live-It meat, and remember: red meat no more than three times a week!

Choose lean cuts of meat and avoid cuts with lots of streaks of white in them. Go for shoulder, rump, chuck, or eye of round. Maybe once in a while a T-bone, a sirloin, or a rib steak—but not too often!

The leanest part of the lamb is the leg, the lamb steak, or the sirloin chop. Somewhat fattier are the loin, rib, shoulder chop, and the shank.

Avoid all pork products completely. A snitch of bacon or a bite of sausage won't kill you (on your birthday!) but don't eat pork products as part of your regular food plan—they're just too fatty.

Non-Live-It Meats you should avoid whenever possible:

all pork	packaged luncheon
ground lamb	meats
regular hamburger	organ meats
duck	(except liver)
goose	frankfurters
	rib steaks

Live-It Fish Isn't Fishy: If you want to have a long, healthy, and lean life, I suggest you meet several fish in the near future. Fish is great for you. Now, I don't mean those fried fish sticks that they used to serve on Fridays in the school cafeteria that you drown in tartar sauce and ketchup and lemon juice after you poked through them with a fork, searching for bones. I'm talking about nice fresh fish that is prepared simply and will make

HOW TO STORE

Don't you just hate it? You're psyched and ready for the best salad of your life. You've spent a half hour soaking in a hot bubble bath, fantasizing the right combination of vegetables, cheeses, and nuts to make a healthy Live-It meal, and then you open the refrigerator and find the lettuce is frozen to the rear side of your Whirlpool Frost-Free. It takes a crowbar to loosen the lettuce, which you finally do about twenty minutes later (after you've lost your appetite from disgust), and then you find that you have to dump about half the lettuce leaves because they are clear green, transparent with ice, and slightly soggy. The mushrooms have shriveled to mouse turds and the cheese has green mold growing on it. And everything was wrapped in plastic!

Where did you go wrong?

Well, let me tell you. There happens to be an art to storing vegetables, and if you expect to Live-It happily ever after with the salads in your life, you'd better run right out and buy yourself one of those highlighting pens for this section of the book.

Lettuce: Store lettuce in a crisper. I don't mean that bottom shelf of the refrigerator that keeps jumping out of the track every time you clean down there; I mean a plastic $4.99 lettuce crisper you buy at the grocery store, the dime store, or the next Tupperware party you happen to go to. With the high price of lettuce these days, you don't want to waste any green stuff on this greenery.

Mushrooms: Mushrooms need air to

your body smile—inside and out. Of course, there are a few fishy exceptions to this rule, so please watch out for sardines, caviar, canned tuna packed in oil, and canned salmon. You can substitute shell-fish for meat in your food plan except for shrimp, which should only be eaten occasionally (and fried shrimp even less occasionally).

A Pause for Pasta: People are always asking my opinion of pasta and the new fad pasta diets. Well, I have a very simple opinion of pasta. I love it. You can't live in Italy all the years I did and not come away as the Spaghetti King. And it's a funny thing about pasta, but it's one of those foods that almost everyone loves. Even kids who won't eat anything else will eat pasta. And pasta, bless its heart,

loves you back. It has a lot of protein in it and is a great energy food. You just have to be real careful not to eat too much of it. Vegetable and whole wheat pastas are the ones I recommend, and those should be eaten in moderation and prior to heavy exercise. *Do not* eat a plate of cannelloni, an entire baking dish of lasagna, and some linguine with red clam sauce and then drink a few beers, watch the ball game, and sack out.

Eggs Are Eggsciting: I'm not one of those people who will tell you never to eat a real egg again in your life. I just want you to know how to count. Don't eat a lot of eggs and never eat eggs for two different meals in the same day. Eggs give great food value for the price and should be included in your food plan.

VEGETABLES

breathe or they will grow mushy and yucky and make you absolutely nauscous just to look at them. Do not put them in plastic Baggies without air! Do keep them in closed brown paper bags in the refrigerator. If you leave them in their cute little baskets or cartons, they won't get yucky but they will shrivel up and begin to look like witches' faces. And lose all their nutrients, too.

Parsley: Parsley is one of those things that you get a whole lot of for not much money, but you don't use so often that you can ever finish off a bunch. So it ends up turning to slime in a plastic Baggie in the pit of your vegetable bin. No more! Freeze parsley. (Sage and rosemary, too, if you like. And thyme. Why not?) Keep the parsley bunch loose and snip off a few

leaves as you need it. It defrosts very quickly!

Potatoes: Do not store potatoes in the fridge because the starch will turn to sugar, the potatoes will get more mealy tasting, and you will be very unhappy when you decide to treat yourself (one medium potato with just a dab of sour cream and butter, remember?). Do keep potatoes in a cool dark place where they can breathe.

Onions: Onions are a lot like potatoes: They will turn to mush in the refrigerator. Store them in a brown paper bag in a cool dry place.

Carrots and Celery: Carrots and celery should be kept in the refrigerator. If they happen to get limp, cut off the ends and stick them in cold water, and they'll crisp right up again.

The Live-It Fruits and Vegetables: Many people think that fruits and vegetables are so good for you that they can eat unlimited quantities whenever they feel like it. They think that instead of having a Danish for a snack, they should have a peach or two and they're being strict with themselves. That's peachy—but it's wrong. Peaches—and all fruits—have natural sugar in them, and sugar is sugar. So, to begin with, don't snack, and don't eat fruit at night. Your Live-It vegetables (avocado is a fruit not a vegetable!) should be steamed—not boiled—if you want them cooked, but can often be eaten raw in salads. And yes, you can have a potato every now and then. Just make sure it's a medium-sized potato and don't fill it up with butter, sour cream, chives, cheese, and crumbled bacon.

Dear Dairy Products: Some people think that the only way to loose weight is to subsist on cottage cheese. Well, I've got news for you. You can eat cottage cheese for the next twenty years, three times a day, and still not have the figure and self-image you're searching for. There's nothing wrong with cottage cheese, and if you like it, eat it and cook with it (the low-fat kind, please). But I don't want you to think that cottage cheese is the key to your salvation. When choosing dairy products for your family and friends, always get the simplest and plainest variety. Buy low-fat or nonfat only. If you're buying yogurt, don't think the raspberry tutti-frutti is going to be as good for you as the 99% fat-free plain version. I suggest you use real butter rather than margarine, but that's up to you. I just would rather have a smidgen of the real thing than some chemicals from a test tube. But don't cook with butter. If you're in need of an ice cream treat, try ice milk. When choosing milk for your coffee, avoid half-and-half, cream, and chemical substitutes and stick to low-fat or nonfat brands. Use yogurt in recipes that call for sour cream and lay back on the processed cheeses and cream cheese—consider them special treats.

Your Live-It Condiments: Despite the fact that there was a short-lived government proclamation that made ketchup a vegetable, I'd like to say I think ketchup is a condiment—one you shouldn't use too often. Don't get me wrong, a little of anything won't hurt you. But some people actually drown their food in ketchup or other such condiments. They say they don't like the taste of a certain food unless it's got ketchup on it, but the simple fact is, they haven't tasted the real food in years—if ever—because the ketchup is all that penetrates their taste buds. If you're looking for more flavor in meats, try marinating them. Don't put salt on anything without tasting it, and try to live without salt at all. Salt is caca, there's no question about it. When you're looking for a cooking oil, go for peanut, safflower, sunflower, walnut, soy, or corn oil—a polyunsaturated vegetable oil. And avoid the use of solid vegetable shortenings.

Your Live-It specialty items: There are a couple of foods that don't seem to fit into any category but are used in many of my recipes and should be part of your real life that I want you to know about. Most of them sound weird but are available in regular grocery stores—look in the gourmet section or the low-sodium section if you don't find them right away. And if your market doesn't carry these products, talk to the manager. Tell him you'll move yourself, your six children, and your mother-in-law into the frozen-foods section of his store (in the heated tent you plan to pitch there) until he thinks of your waistline.

TAMARI:

A brown soy sauce–like liquid with a lot less salt than soy sauce. Buy also at health food stores.

MILD SOY SAUCE:

You've heard of light beer? Well, this is mild soy sauce with about half the salt of the regular variety. We found it in the grocery store next to the old fashioned kind.

SESAME SEEDS:

I like them roasted to add a little extra crunch to a dish.

BULGAR WHEAT:

Buy at health food stores if your grocery doesn't stock, and use like rice. It has a faster cooking time than rice, is a lot more nutritional, and has a nuttier flavor, too. Use in salads, soups, casseroles, even for cous cous.

DRY MUSTARD:

Why use the water-based chemical mustard when you can use dried from the spice rack? It's especially good in meals that need no additional liquid additives. Also great in salad dressings. And a little goes a long way.

NEUFCHÂTEL CHEESE:

If it looks like cream cheese and comes in a package like cream cheese, it must be Neufchâtel cheese. Try it on a bagel or in recipes that call for cream cheese or sour cream. Not so good on a baked potato.

SHALLOTS, SCALLIONS, AND SCALLOPS:

I keep getting these three things mixed up, so if you do, too, here goes:

Shallots are small onionlike bulbs that are great for adding flavor.

Scallions also add flavor. They're green onions and you can cut them up with a scissors and snip into salads or meals.

Scallops are shellfish and have nothing at all to do with onions.

MEET YOUR LIVE-IT KITCHEN

When you decided to start your life over and live it the Live-It way, you made an important decision that involved a lot of discipline. If you've lost weight on the Live-It, I know you've got the discipline you need to be successful in everything you do. So I've got something new for you to do. You've already reorganized your day, right? Now I want you to reorganize your kitchen.

The kitchen has several enemies of the overweight lurking in the most inconspicuous places. You've got to know where to look for them and you've got to know how to destroy them—before they get to you. Remember *The Exorcist*? Well now, we're going to purge your kitchen of the tools of the Devil. And we're also going to make some new friends in there.

So get up, shut off the television set, and carry this book into the kitchen. Stand facing the sink and then begin reading again. We're going to work our way around the room.

This is your sink. Your sink is your friend. You wash your fruits and veggies here. The sink is your baptismal font where you will start your Live-It life anew. And because you're going to be eating many more fruits and vegetables than you used to, you're going to get very well-acquainted with your sink.

This is your stove. What you're used to seeing on your stove is a teapot and three frying pans. Kiss those frying pans good-bye and reintroduce yourself to your stove. Now that you're on the Live-It, you'll be using steamers for vegetables and fish and stir-frying in a wok—not French frying or sautéeing in butter and garlic. So bury your frying pans in a box in the garage. Treat yourself to a steamer and get used to the new look your stove has taken on.

This is your refrigerator. Your refrigerator is a double agent—it can be friend or foe, depending on you. Stock it with fresh healthful foods and clean it regularly. You weigh yourself every morning, right? Well, clean your refrigerator twice a week. And do it *after* a meal, not before

one. Let's just take a peek in your fridge right now so you can see what I'm talking about. Now, I know you're not a slob and you clean the icebox once a week. But there's a big difference between cleaning to get out the smells and cleaning to help yourself keep weight off. So here's the Live-It tour of your refrigerator.

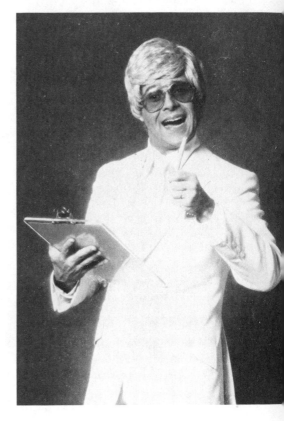

"Hi there, folks, I'm your tour guide, Doug. Welcome aboard. Right here we have a [fill in your own brand name here] refrigerator; she sure is a beauty. A full sixteen-point-four cubic feet of cooled air. Let's open the door and take a look inside. Uh-huh, look at that: a half a head of lettuce wrapped in cellophane and frozen to the side of the refrigerator; ten Tupperware containers, unmarked, filled with mystery ingredients. All over two days old. There's half a bottle of flat club soda—tastes great like that, doesn't it?—and some tomato juice still in the can. Whatcha going to mix that with later on in the day? There's a few dried-up lemons, quite a large selection of jams and jellies, and oh, my goodness, do we have a not quite full can of olives right here?

"Now, let's look up in the freezer. Oh my God, no! Frozen Milky Ways? Three different kinds of ice cream? A Sara Lee pound cake? Hawaiian Punch popsicles? I can't believe my eyes. TV dinners?

"Well, excuse me, folks, we've obviously taken you into an X-rated freezer. We thought the owner of this refrigerator was on the Live-It."

Okay, now that we know what's behind the white door, let's get in there and clean up. Put down this book immediately and bring out a sponge and cleaning foam. Throw out anything that's been in the refrigerator for more than four days unless it's a packaged condiment (e.g., ketchup, mustard, jam, etc.). Get rid of the tinfoil swan, the paper carton of Chinese food, the bent-out-of-shape container of pineapple rings. Now, dip that sponge and scrub those glass shelves. Keep repeating to yourself, "I promise

not to befoul my fridge ever again." Rinse and blow-dry. (Just kidding.) There's going to be inspection, so stand at attention until your counselor excuses you for recess.

This is your food processor. When the Cuisinart was first introduced in this country, I thought it was so important, I bought dozens of them wholesale and sold them at that price to the people who exercised at the Anatomy Asylum. Now anyone can afford to buy a food processor because they sell them for $34.95, and they do everything but tap-dance. It's not essential to own a food processor. I wouldn't tell you to go out and get an extra job to raise the money to buy one. But I think that for thirty-five bucks it buys you an awful lot of convenience. You'll be saved the boredom of chopping and dicing, and you'll have quick and easy-to-reach-for foods that are healthful rather than sugar-filled. Salads and vegetables are important for a person who is giving up fattening foods, and the food processor does help you vary your meals with a minimum of trouble.

This is your set of separate measuring cups. Measuring cups come in many shapes and varieties. You can get that giant Pyrex measuring cup with the seven thousand red lines on it that will serve every purpose in your life and consider yourself equipped forever. Or you can get smart and buy yourself a set of separate measuring cups with one for each size. Yes, they take up more room. Yes, you can always lose one (or several) of the individual cups. Yes, it's more work if you move and you have to pack everything yourself. *BUT* you'll never add too much of any ingredient. And that's definitely worth $1.39.

This is your Mixmaster. My, what a pretty Mixmaster. I was sure you'd have a relatively new, high-powered, fancy-shmancy Mixmaster instead of one of those little portable jobs. Got it for Christmas or your birthday, right? Well, now there's something you can get for your Mixmaster. A combination lock. And let someone else keep the combination. On your Live-It you will rarely need a Mixmaster, especially if you've got a food processor. Let's face it, kids: You just aren't going to be making too many more lemon meringue pies.

This is your blender. You know your blender—you've made milk shakes and ice cream sodas in it in the middle of the night when you needed a friend and something to wash down those brownies you were munching on. You even got a silent *whirrrr* kind of blender so you wouldn't wake up the whole house with your missions at midnight. Well, now it's time for a little behavior modification. You can still use your blender on your Live-It plan, but never in the middle of the night. You can still use your blender, but for making protein drinks and soups, not for ice cream snacks. Since changing behavior is a matter of changing habits, I have a little project for you. Place a few tomatoes and cucumbers in your blender at night. Don't turn on the blender; just let them sit there. If you get up in the middle of the night for a shake, you'll discover the ingredients for a cup of gazpacho. You can make gazpacho, then put it in the refrigerator to chill or you can take the veggies and put them back in the fridge and go back to bed.

MEET YOUR LIVE-IT BODY

Remember the ninety-seven-pound weakling whose entire life was dedicated to becoming Superman? He was the guy in the back of the classroom with the thick glasses, the slide rule in a plastic case attached to his belt, and his hand always waving in the air to answer the teacher's question before she finished the sentence. Invariably he was short, pimply, and skinny. And all he wanted to be was tall, muscular, and gorgeous.

Me too. Except I was the fat kid in the front row always making the jokes and getting everyone to laugh and have fun when they were supposed to be naming the tributaries of the Mississippi River. I, too, had a dream. That I would someday be tall and muscular and gorgeous.

Well, I haven't figured out the tall part yet. I mean, you just can't do too much to change your height. But other than that, you can change every other part of your body. I know, because I did it. Your skeleton is yours. The rest is in your hands and in your mind.

You can trade in your pudgy, sagging, and not too petite frame for a new model—complete with sunroof and wire wheels. In fact, no food plan is going to work for you unless you are willing to give up your old body. I'm not talking about repairs here, I'm talking about an overhaul. Why? Because of all the people in this entire huge gigantic country who have been on diets, the only ones who keep the weight off permanently are the ones who have a rigorous exercise program. Exercise is not only the key to keeping the fat off, it's the whole secret to keeping the good looks going.

And let's face it, we all want to be better-looking.

So the Live-It body is the changing body. The weight is coming off, the chins are disappearing, the arms are slimming down, the hips are getting narrower and narrower, and the head is being held up higher and higher because of the pride you have in your new body.

The Live-It body is on its way to becoming firm, healthy, and taut with power. The Live-It body is on its way to longer life and maintained happiness because it can do things a fat body can't do; it can attract people and jobs a fat body can't; and it can increase the owner's self-confidence. (Do you own your body? Well, if you don't, no one else can, right?) And with self-confidence we can do anything.

YOUR LIVE-IT MIND

No one, I mean absolutely no one, is going to lose weight without wanting to. And without working for it. As much as we would all like to pray to the Weight Loss Fairy to come and take away our extra poundage while we sleep, it just doesn't work that way.

Losing weight, and keeping weight off, is neither simple nor easy.

It's hard, hard work. And don't believe anyone who tells you anything else.

Yet, there are people who have lost weight and who have complete control over their figures. How do they do it? What is their trick?

It's all in the mind.

When you make up your mind to get on a sensible food plan and a healthful exercise program and to stick to them until you reach your goal, you can accomplish anything. And once you begin to lose weight and see your life change, you'll know that no one can stop you.

You have the power to be the best *you* possible. You can be as beautiful outside as you are inside. It's hard, and sometimes it hurts. But it's worth it, I think.

I'm here to hold your hand and help you through it.

Together we can do it. Together we can do anything.

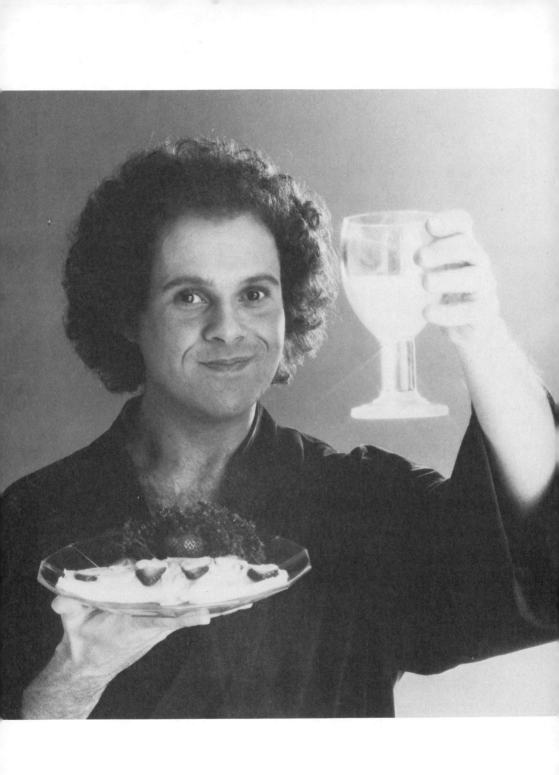

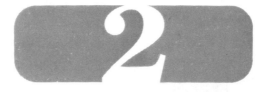

Morning Becomes Electric

THE BREAKFAST PLEDGE

Take the Breakfast Pledge each morning while looking in the mirror.

Good morning, _____ (fill in your name). Well, you're starting a brand-new day, and something you should be thinking about right this very moment is that you haven't gained any weight yet today. And it's already _____ (fill in exact time). I'm proud of you!

Now, I know you are not, I repeat, *not*, going in that kitchen to nibble on _____ (fill in last night's leftovers). Nor will you be taking a quick peek in the freezer to get out something for tonight's dinner while you help yourself to a few bites of _____ (you know what it is you keep in the freezer that no one else knows about). No, not today. You're not going to start another day like that.

(Pause here for one moment to softly pinch your cheek.)

Now, raise your right arm and take the Breakfast Pledge.

I solemnly swear to have a nutritious vitamin-filled breakfast, to avoid all fads and phony foods, and to stick to my Live-It program. So help me God. Amen.

Congratulations and good morning.

THE MORNING BLUES

There are people in this world who jump out of bed each morning with bright eyes, clear heads, and veins pulsating with adrenaline. They don't need a cup of coffee to wake them up because they are already singing to the birds (usually off-key—but the birds never notice) and hurriedly doing their own thing as if they were on a drug high. This is one out of every 614,000 persons in the world, but there are people like that.

Then there are people who let the alarm clock ring for a full three minutes before throwing it against the wall and falling back asleep. They needn't worry about being late for work or school because they already know they would never naturally wake up before noon, so they've set up a fail-safe system for themselves. Five minutes after the first alarm, another alarm rings from across the room. This alarm is usually ignored with a drowsy shrug. In another five minutes several clocks begin to chime. There's an electronic robot clock that actually speaks English and says, "Good morning. It's eight fifteen." There's a clock with lasers set into it that sends blinding light to the eyes so these people have to get out of bed just to escape the glare. There's a clock that emulates sunrise and throws an orange hue across the bedroom. This one comes complete with its own shovel that will actually toss them from bed to bathroom. There they can shower, shave, dress, and get on with the day without being awake.

Granted, both of these types are ex-tremes, and there are millions of people who fall somewhere in between. They get up in the morning because they have obligations, and they work their way through a morning of mazes because they have no other choices. Some people actually do function better in the morning, and some people really are night people. But with society structured the way it is and the workday based on the clock rather than individual biology, people have few choices but to face the morning hours and bear them as gracefully as possible.

But a bad start in the morning can mean a bad day. And there's no reason to let yourself in for the kind of aggravation you can actually avoid. You don't have to bumble blindly through the day until noon. You needn't be a grouch until an intravenous infusion of coffee comes your way. And you needn't be one of those rare early birds who crows at sunrise either. Each person has his own morning I.Q., and even if you are a night person, there are ways to ease yourself into morning that will make your day just a little bit better.

So let's take this quiz and figure out exactly what your morning profile is. Then we'll give you a breakfast plan that will keep you on your Live-It and still make you a happy person. Mother was right. Breakfast is the most important meal of the day, and no matter how you wake up in the morning, there's a breakfast that's right for you. So answer these questions, please. There's no right or wrong answer, so this isn't anything you have to pass or fail. Just do me one favor. If you're not a morning person, take this test at night!

THE BREAKFAST QUIZ

1. When I wake up in the morning:
a. I check the alarm clock, look out the window, turn on the radio or TV, and spend a few seconds thinking about my day.
b. I roll over and go back to sleep again.
c. I bound out of bed filled with energy and good cheer.

2. The first thing I do after opening my eyes is:
a. turn on the television or radio.
b. Who can remember?
c. begin worrying about my busy schedule.

3. For breakfast I:
a. have a simple meal while reading the newspaper or watching TV.
b. never eat; I haven't got time.
c. never eat; breakfast makes me whoops.

4. If there were no time pressures in the morning, my ideal breakfast would be:
a. eggs, toast, and bacon; eaten sensibly in the kitchen.
b. breakfast in bed on a white wicker tray—maybe some eggs, croissants, jam, and butter, with a big china pot of steaming coffee. And don't forget the red rosebud.
c. none at all; I already told you, breakfast makes me sick.

5. My morning routine includes:
a. shower, news source, family time, makeup, and dress for the day's activities.
b. shower, several cups of coffee, and a newspaper to read on the way out the door.
c. brushing my teeth, throwing on my clothes, and getting out of the house as fast as possible.

6. I think that exercise in the morning:
a. is a great idea that I always try to incorporate in my life-style.
b. makes me feel better when I take time to do it.
c. is a waste of time. I get plenty of exercise during the day.

7. If I had an especially busy day lined up, in order to fit everything in I would:
a. get up a half hour earlier that morning; stay up a half hour later that night.
b. stay up all night until I was finished.
c. get up at dawn and get cracking.

8. I get all my best ideas:
a. driving along a peaceful road.
b. late at night or as I'm falling asleep.
c. in the shower, first thing in the morning.

9. **I think that breakfast is:**
a. the most important meal of the day.
b. a nice luxury.
c. a waste of time.

10. **My favorite meal of the day is:**
a. breakfast.
b. dinner.
c. lunch.

Before you begin to score this quiz, I think there's something you should know about it. This quiz is rigged. There are no right or wrong answers. So if you circled an answer because you thought it was right, and you were afraid you'd flunk out right here in the second chapter, go back now and set the record straight. This is a profile quiz, and chances are, most of your answers are the same letters, because morning patterns break down into three distinctly different types of people.

If you have mostly (a) answers

Congratulations, you're just about as normal as can be. You could use a little more discipline in your morning routine and you've got to start exercising regularly, but you are a steady, average, normal person. Your typical breakfast menu should look like this:

1 cup of herb tea
1 glass of juice or one piece of fresh fruit (not both)
Live-It-Up Danish (See Live-It recipe p. 50) or Quickie Breakfast Quiche (See p. 83) or 1 egg

If you have mostly (b) answers

You're a night person, pure and simple. You hate mornings and function best after four P.M. in the afternoon. You have a tendency to begin weight-loss programs and then toss them aside because they don't fit your life-style. If it were up to you, you'd totally abolish morning and would begin the workday at noon. You're going to need a good bit of training in behavior modification to learn to conquer mornings and eat a proper breakfast.

Your typical breakfast menu should look like this:

½ cup of coffee with ½ cup skim or low-fat milk (No sugar, please.)
1 piece of fresh fruit, preferably cold enough to wake up your teeth, or Fresh Fruit Cup (See Live-It recipe for Fresh Fruit Cups, p. 47.)
1 bowl of cereal(without fruit in it)

You want to keep your breakfast light, and let exercise help wake you up rather than caffeine or sugar. You're the type of person who grabs a doughnut at the office or eats a container of Sara Lee sweet rolls while drinking cup after cup of coffee, so knock it off. You can gain five pounds before you're fully awake. Exercise is the answer to your problems. Honest.

If you have mostly (c) answers

One in 614,000, I finally found you! You are a true morning person and are totally misunderstood by most of your fellow human beings. Your body is going at 90 mph when you wake up, and you have no patience for exercise or breakfast or anything that gets in your way or slows you down. All you want to do is conquer the world—immediately. Well, that's fine. But, c'mon, admit it. Don't you fall apart at four in the afternoon? I am just going to have to show you how to live a little longer—and a little better.

◎◎◎◎

When you do your morning stretches and exercises, concentrate on going slowly and breathing properly between each set. Don't bound through them as if you were a racehorse setting a time trial. Handle breakfast the same way—slow and steady wins the race. Your breakfast will be light, but it's important to eat it. Your typical breakfast menu should look something like this:

1 8-ounce glass warm water with 1 to 2 teaspoons lemon juice
1 4-ounce glass of juice (Avoid citrus juices.)
1 slice whole wheat toast or ½ whole wheat muffin, with 1 pat of butter
1 scrambled egg

In scoring, remember that these are body types, not right or wrong scores. It doesn't matter which style you came out. But you do need to know, especially if you've been skipping breakfast. The typical menu listed in each category is just to give you a general idea of proportions and what breakfast should look and feel like. If you eat eggs Monday, you prob-ably won't want eggs Tuesday. So don't get rigid about the menu I just listed. And this is a cookbook, so you can experiment. Just remember that (b) and (c) profiles should try to go light, and (a) should hold back from too much.

EXERCISE AND STRETCH SCHEDULE

Good morning. Here is your morning exercise and stretch schedule. If you have trouble opening your eyes to read it in the morning, read it at night before you go to bed.

These exercises and stretches are for men, women, and children of any weight. If you have never exercised before, consult a doctor before you begin this schedule. If you need to lose a tremendous amount of weight, these exercises are in addition to your regular morning routine. (And don't worry, we'll be adding to your evening schedule as well.) These exercises and stretches have been devised to get you revved up and ready to conquer the day. They are not strenuous enough to create a weight loss—especially after you binged out last night on linguine and clam sauce. These exercises are mostly for circulation and toning. So if you have a serious weight problem, don't think these exercises are your ticket to easy street. If you are maintaining a weight loss and you follow the food and exercise instructions in this book, you should not need any additional exercise program. But you shouldn't break your Live-It either.

Okay, here goes.

Good morning everyone.

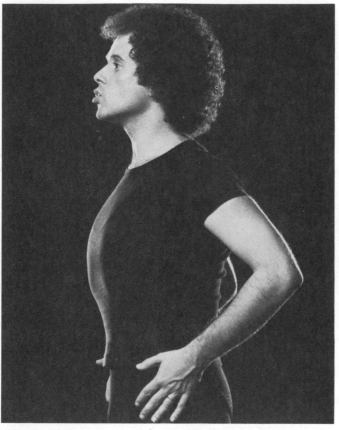

Deep Breathing
5 deep inhales; 5 deep exhales

Stand up straight, neck up, and:
1. Inhale through your nose (keep going, keep going, keep going, that's it!).
2. Keep that air in for the count of 100—just kidding. Hold for a count of five:

| ONE | THREE | FIVE |
| TWO | FOUR | |

3. Let out the air slowly, hold your stomach in, and relax. Good.

Keep your stomach in, stand up straight, chin in.

1. Place your hands on your lower stomach—below the belly button.
2. Inhale a lot of air through your nose.
3. Slowly let the air out of your mouth and at the same time press gently on your tum. Keep pressing until you release as much air as possible. Blow it out. Let me hear you.

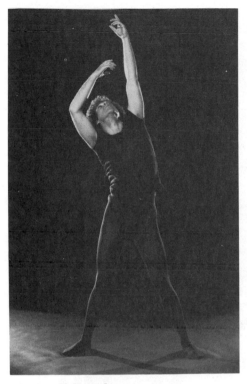 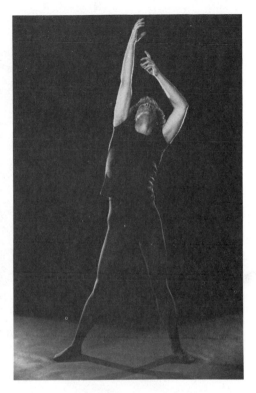

Climb and Stretch
30 climbs, 15 each hand

● Stay in your standing position, feet apart. Hold your stomach in, lift your neck high, and look at the ceiling.

● Bring both hands above the head as if you're ready to climb a rope. Alternate your breathing as you shift your upper torso. Right-hand reach as you *inhale*, left-hand reach as you *exhale*.

● You should feel all the pulling sensation in your shoulders and also from your waist (keep that stomach in, and tight).

● Just keep thinking about pulling that rope higher and higher. Come on, it's a rope, not a piece of dental floss.

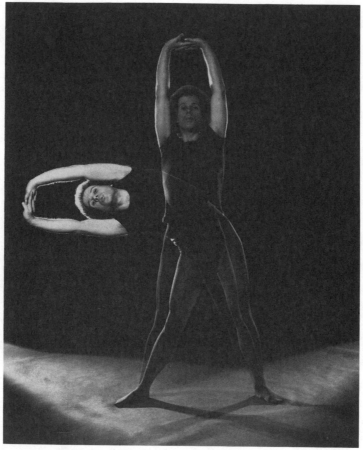

Side Bends
30 bends, 15 right; 15 left

Side Bends

● Same position. This time lace your fingers together, elbows nice and straight, head up—stomach in.

● Inhale (through your nose) and S-L-O-W-L-Y exhale as you bend all the way to the left. Don't worry how low you can bend—it may take a while for your muscles to respond; besides, we know there's cheesecake or root-

beer floats stored somewhere between your ribcage and your hip.

● Inhale as you S-L-O-W-L-Y take up the upper part of your body and repeat on the right side.

● These bends not only limber up your sides but also stretch your arms, chest, back, and neck areas.

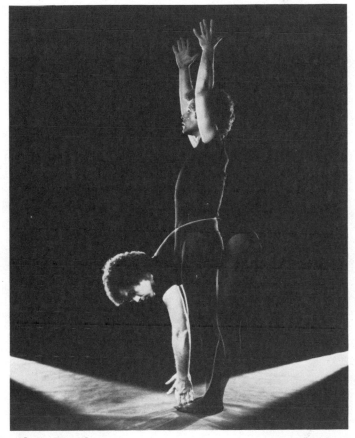

Back and Vertebrae Stretch
10, all the way to the toes

Back and Vertebrae Stretch
• Legs together please, stomach in, tighten your rear, and check your neck (always keep that chin up).

• Again, bring both hands over your head and spread your fingers wide—they need some air and exercise, too.

• Inhale and S-L-O-W-L-Y exhale as you begin your descent to your toes area. Now hold that stomach in. Inhale on the way back up and exhale as you go down again.

• This exercise stretches your whole back side—neck, shoulders, vertebrae, back, and legs. The muscles in your legs may be tight and getting all the way to the toes may seem impossible. Don't worry—they'll loosen up and stay firm.

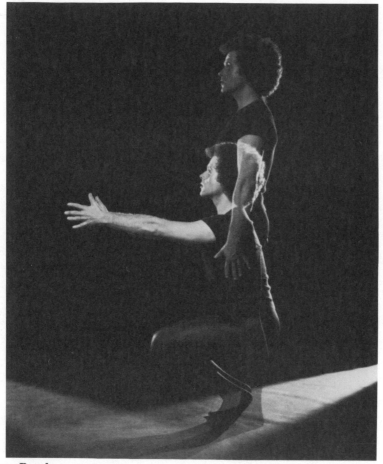

Deep Knee Bends
5 bends, through the legs, please

Deep-Knee Bends

● Now it's time to stretch your knees and the front and inside of your legs.

● Feet apart, give me your best posture. Come on, just think what that body of yours is gonna look like soon. Get those arms up above your head.

● Inhale and as you exhale bend your knees and take a dive between your legs pushing both hands through the leg opening. (Like Esther Williams in *Summer in the Everglades.*)

● Inhale and come up again, exhale and swing down there, keeping that stomach in tight. (Remember also to round your neck and head and to do these nice for Esther!)

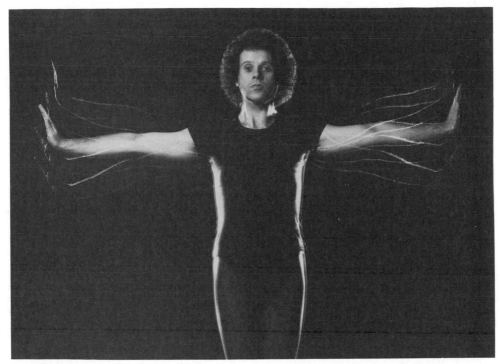

Arm Circles
15 each way

Arm Circles

● Legs tight, real tight, please. Chin up and smile. We're gonna make those arms slim and tight so that when you wave to someone your whole arm doesn't jiggle around like a dish of Jell-O.

● Extend both arms, tighten them, and flatten the palms of your hands.

● Begin rotating your arms, at first with small circles, then working up to bigger ones. Keep a constant flow of air circulating through the lungs. Inhale through nose, exhale through mouth. Don't do this exercise to real fast music or you'll find yourself flying out the window.

● Remember, clockwise and counterclockwise.

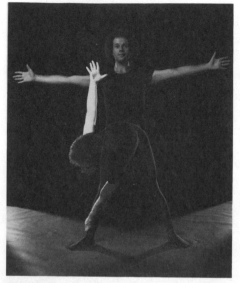 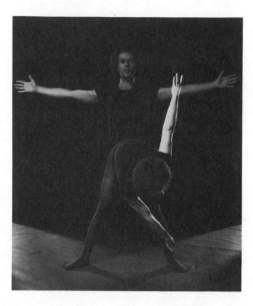

Toe to Toe
30 turns, 15 each direction

● Spread your feet wide. S-L-O-W-L-Y bend down as if you're removing gum from the front of your shoe.

● With your left hand touch your right foot and inhale. Switch, and now exhale as your right hand touches your left foot.

● Stay down low and keep switching from left to right.

● Remember to keep the other arm high in the air, so while one arm is stretching down the other is stretching up—that's real balance.

● This is the greatest exercise for your waistline, hips, and thighs, and also helps firm up the arms.

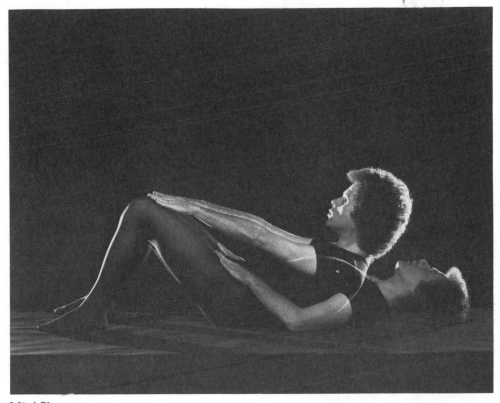

Mini Sit-ups
20

● Lie down on the floor. (No, this is not a rest period—this is tummy period.) Bend your knees and spread your feet a bit.

● Rest your hands at the base of your legs. Inhale with your back and head flat on the floor. Exhale while you slowly glide up your legs all the way to your knee caps. Keep your chin tucked into your chest. Inhale as you go down.

● Believe me, this one is a killer at first. The thing this exercise does right away is make you aware of the fat around your stomach. You put it there and only you can get rid of it. And you will, I promise you. Now that news is something to sit up about! Remember, the slower you do these the more your fat cells will hate you.

Good for you! Now, don't you feel better?

YOUR MORNING SCHEDULE

If you're one of those people who is so catatonic in the morning that you need someone to point you in the right direction and get you going on the right path to life, I've come up with a little helping hand. Here is a morning schedule for you.

All you need to follow it is to know how to read. Just cut out whichever of these two schedules pertains to your life-style (one for people who work, one for people who don't) and tape it to the lamp on your side of the bed. Then, after you wake up, pull yourself up toward the light and read off your list of instructions. In no time at all you'll be energized and ready to tackle the world.

----------*IF YOU WORK OUT OF THE HOUSE*----------

7:00: Wake up. All right, everybody, rise and shine.

7:05: Second wake-up. All right, everybody, I said rise and shine. Get with it.

7:08: So all right already. Get your tush moving. I want you up, on your feet, and doing your stretch exercises.

7:10: That's right, it's time to exercise. Stay in your nightgown or jammies, it's okay. If you want to go out and buy a lemon-yellow leotard in cotton-stretch Spandex nylon with double crotch and wire wheels for this part of the morning, that's your business. But you can do these stretches naked, as far as I'm concerned.

7:30: Head for the bathroom now. Time to brush your teeth, shower, shave, plug in the electric rollers, and dress. (Your clothes should have been picked out the day before—it saves time and decisions in the morning. And don't wear what you wore yesterday—it's bad for morale.)

8:00: Your Live-It breakfast. (Consult your breakfast plan, your Live-It volume food plan in *Never-Say-Diet*, and the recipes in this chapter.)

8:30: Leave home.

9:00: Arrive at office.

9:05: Arrive at office. Okay, okay, so you left the house a little late. Or you needed gas. No one's perfect.

---*IF YOU STAY HOME*---

6:30: Wake up to sound of kids fighting. Roll over and groan.

6:35: Admit that you can't get back to sleep so you might as well get up.

6:37: Tell spouse "Not now."

6:45: Stop kids from killing each other while you try to brush your teeth.

6:47: Try to brush your teeth again, praying for silence in the house.

6:50: Feed cats, dog, goldfish. Line up kids with you for morning stretches.

7:10: Send kids to get dressed (matching clothes laid out from night before) while you shower quickly.

7:15: Head for kitchen while kids finish dressing. Sort out lunches for school children and prepare breakfast for family.

7:25: Serve breakfast to family at the breakfast table.

7:45: Drive car pool.

8:15: Return from car pool. Sit down to a cup of hot water and lemon juice or herb tea and have five minutes of quiet time for yourself. This is no time for coffee, so forget it right now. Make up your shopping list, write down your errands for the day and your projects to get done.

8:30: Begin kitchen cleanup and bed making.

9:00: Ready to watch *The Richard Simmons Show*?

THE CLEAN UP AND CLEAR UP CHECKLIST

It's that time of day. The hubby's gone to work. The kids are off to school, or at least they're out playing in the yard. You're alone with just a morning news-program to cheer you up and the sight of the breakfast table to bring zip into your morning.

What? The sight of the breakfast table isn't so inspiring after all? Well, let's take a look and see what you've got there. Maybe you and your family are eating the wrong things for breakfast. Pull out a pencil and take this book over to the table (uncleared table, of course) and just check off the things that apply to your mess. If you've already cleared the table, not to worry. Just move to the sink and sort out that pile of sticky dishes. You can't fool me. I knew you were saving those dishes for later. You wanted the grease to soak off in hot water, right?

C'mon, let's see what you're hiding under that ring around your sink.

_____ sticky, gooey golden remnants of maple syrup

_____ breakfast-sausage tidbits (links or patties, no difference)

_____ leftover bacon strips

_____ pats of butter or margarine, now dumped to the side of the plate

_____ dirty coffee cups

_____ creamer that contained half-and-half

_____ tinfoil container that sweet rolls were in (You plan to wash and save container.)

_____ sugar-coated, now soggy, cereal bits

_____ pizza crusts

_____ avocado and sour cream dabbles

_____ confectioner's sugar stuck to Grand Marnier sauce

_____ raisins and pecans, signifying the previous existence of a coffee cake.

Let's take a look at how many of these you have marked. Oh, no! Shame on you. Two marks, I would have thought I was teaching you a little something. But all those? Just tell me how you expect to lose weight when you eat like that? And how do you expect your family to grow up healthy with all that disgusting sweet food in the house? You better put masking tape around your waffle iron right now. Go to the cupboard and grab that maple syrup and throw it away. (Don't give it to the Salvation Army, they don't need it either.) You better get down on your hands and knees and pray for guidance and willpower, because you're in terrible trouble. Coffee cakes! Prepackaged sweet rolls! Sour cream and avocado omelets! No wonder you have hotcake hips.

Well, my friend, those days of overeating are over. I am here to rescue you from yourself. You better get those dishes done now—I mean, right now. And then don't stop and come back to this book. I don't want you to pick up this book until you've cleaned your cupboards as well. I don't happen to believe too much in torture, so let yourself off easy. Why have these fattening foods in your home if you can't eat them? The rest of your family doesn't need them any more than you do. Take control and clean up and clear out. Now. I'll wait right here. You get going.

SPECIALTY BREAKFASTS

Let's face it. There are times when breakfast is more than the most important meal of the day. It's a social occasion, a business occasion or even a celebration. You may be on vacation. Your parents may be visiting. You just may be in the mood for a break in your usual routine. Can one still lose weight and have a luxurious breakfast? Absolutely.

We've taken six of the world's most famous breakfast dishes and converted them to the metric system. No, no, no. Just kidding there. What we've really done is shown you how to modify a traditional, old-fashioned fattening breakfast into something that's just as terrific but not nearly as fattening. Blintzes can be yours!

That doesn't mean you can dump your old Live-It food plan and substitute any or all of these recipes immediately. These are special-occasion breakfasts. If you have one of them once a week, you'll enjoy the treat and still lose weight.

Eggs Benedict
Forget the hollandaise (and the holland nights) and just enjoy.

Serves Two

1 tablespoon butter	2 eggs
1 tablespoon flour	1 large tomato, sliced thin
½ cup low-fat milk	juice of 1 lemon
¼ cup nonfat dry powdered milk	freshly ground pepper
2 slices whole wheat bread	paprika

1. Melt butter in small saucepan, add flour, and mix until smooth. Combine milks and slowly add to flour, stirring constantly. Remove from heat.
2. Toast bread. Poach eggs by dropping into boiling water and simmering until whites are set.
3. Remove eggs with a skimmer. Drain well. Place half the tomato slices on each piece of toast. Place egg on top.
4. Reheat milk mixture slightly, add lemon juice, and pour over eggs. Sprinkle with pepper and paprika. Serve immediately.

Strawberry Omelet
This one's the berries.

Serves Two

1 cup fresh strawberries	oil
¼ cup yogurt	water
1 squeeze of lemon juice	parsley for garnish
2 eggs	

1. Mash ⅓ cup strawberries with yogurt and lemon juice. Thinly slice remaining strawberries and set aside.
2. Lightly oil 9-inch nonstick skillet by wiping oil on pan with a paper towel. Blend eggs together with a fork, adding a few drops of water.
3. Pour eggs into skillet and cook over medium heat until eggs begin to set. Lift the edges, allowing the unset portion to run underneath by tilting the pan.
4. Place the sliced fruit in the center of the omelet, reserving a few slices for garnish.
5. Using a spatula, gently fold the edges of the omelet into the center.
6. Top with yogurt mixture and garnish with reserved strawberry slices and parsley.

Huevos Rancheros
Olé to you this morning.

Serves Two

2 teaspoons olive oil
½ cup onion, diced
½ green pepper, diced
1 clove garlic, minced

1 cup chopped tomatoes
freshly ground pepper
¼ teaspoon dried crushed basil
2 eggs

1. In medium frying pan, heat oil. Sauté onion and green pepper until onion becomes translucent.
2. Add garlic, tomato, and seasonings. Cook over low heat for 2 minutes, stirring.
3. Make 2 holes in sauce with a spoon and crack eggs in. Cover and cook until eggs are set.

French Apple Toast
Put a little ooh la la in your morning.

Serves Two

2 slices whole wheat bread
2 eggs
¼ cup low-fat milk

½ teaspoon nutmeg
½ teaspoon cinnamon
1 apple, cored and thinly sliced

1. Beat together eggs, milk, and nutmeg in pie plate or small oven tray. Soak bread in mixture until bread is completely saturated.
2. Place apple slices around bread along edge of tray, and sprinkle with cinnamon and nutmeg.
3. Place tray in preheated 375°F oven and bake until bread is puffy and golden brown. Serve each bread slice with half the baked apples.

Eggs Florentine
A tasty trip to Italy without pasta.

Serves Two

1 cup cooked spinach
2 tablespoons low-fat milk mixed with
2 tablespoons nonfat dry powdered milk
freshly ground pepper
nutmeg

2 eggs
2 tablespoons freshly grated Parmesan cheese
2 tablespoons whole wheat bread crumbs
paprika

1. Place half the spinach in individual baking dish. Add half the amount of pepper and nutmeg; add milk mixture to dishes.
2. Make a hollow in center of each dish and carefully crack each egg in.
3. Sprinkle top of each with 1 tablespoon Parmesan cheese and 1 tablespoon bread crumbs. Top with paprika.
4. Bake in preheated 375°F oven until eggs are set.

Cheesy Blintzes

Your grandmother should try these!

Serves Four

Blintzes:
3 eggs
3 tablespoons water
2 tablespoons flour

2 tablespoons nonfat dry powdered milk

Filling:
⅔ cup low-fat cottage cheese
1 egg
¼ cup plain low-fat yogurt
½ teaspoon grated orange rind

1 tablespoon frozen orange juice concentrate
1 teaspoon honey
½ teaspoon vanilla

Topping:
½ cup fresh pineapple
½ cup fresh orange

1 teaspoon arrowroot

1. Beat eggs, water, flour, and powdered milk together.
2. Make crepes by pouring 3 tablespoons of batter into a small (6 inch) nonstick skillet. Tilt skillet to spread batter evenly over bottom.
3. Cook over medium high heat for about 1 minute or until lightly brown on one side. Turn out onto paper towels.
4. Combine filling ingredients in blender until smooth.
5. Place a heaping tablespoon of filling on the browned side of each crepe. Roll up, tucking in ends. Place side by side in small casserole or pie plate.
6. Bake in preheated 300°F oven for 10 to 15 minutes.
7. Puree together pineapple, orange, and arrowroot. Place in small saucepan. Simmer for 3 to 4 minutes. Cool. Serve each blintz with 1 tablespoon topping.

FAST-BREAKING BREAKFASTS

Eggs McSimmons

You deserve a break today.

Serves Two

1 whole wheat English muffin
2 eggs
2 thin slices cooked turkey
2 slices tomato (optional)

2 thin slices sharp Cheddar cheese (4- by 1½-inch pieces)
paprika and parsley for garnish

1. Split muffin in half. Lightly toast both sides.
2. Poach eggs by carefully cracking them into boiling water. Cook until the whites are set.
3. Place 1 slice of turkey on each muffin half. Top with tomato slice and poached egg. Cut cheese slices in half diagonally and place on top of each egg.
4. Run each muffin under broiler for 1 to 2 minutes until cheese melts. Sprinkle with paprika and garnish with parsley.

Ricotta Omelet

You gotta taste the ricotta!

Serves Four

¼ cup chopped cooked chicken or turkey
½ cup fresh diced pineapple
½ cup low-fat ricotta cheese

1 teaspoon butter
3 eggs
2 teaspoons low-fat milk
chopped parsley

1. Combine chicken (or turkey), pineapple, and ricotta cheese.
2. In nonstick pan, melt butter. Beat eggs and milk together and pour into pan. Allow omelet to cook around sides and middle, using medium–low heat.
3. Spread ricotta cheese mixture over eggs. Fold over one side of omelet and continue to cook until eggs are done and not runny.
4. Sprinkle parsley on top of omelet and serve.
   If some cheese mixture oozes out, do not fret—it may be eaten anyway.

From the kitchen of Tracey Lord Lawrence

Pineapple Roll-Up

A trip to Hawaii in every tropical bite.

Serves One

1 slice day-old whole grain bread	½ cup crushed pineapple
1 egg, beaten	¼ teaspoon club soda
1 teaspoon honey	½ teaspoon cinnamon
⅓ cup nonfat dry powdered milk	1 teaspoon butter

1. Crumble bread in blender. Place in small mixing bowl. Add egg, honey, powdered milk, pineapple, soda, cinnamon and butter. Mix well.
2. Place in 8-inch nonstick cake pan. Bake in 375°F oven for 12 to 15 minutes.
3. Roll up like an Enchilada and enjoy.

From the kitchen of Rose Marie Montgomery

Fresh Fruit Cups

Just so your fruit cup doesn't runneth over.

Serves Two

1 cantaloupe	¼ cup finely chopped nuts
½ ripe banana, sliced	½ teaspoon cinnamon
1 orange, peeled and sectioned	fresh mint leaves
4 strawberries	

1. Cut cantaloupe in half and remove seeds. Fill center of each with banana and orange slices.
2. Place 2 strawberries on each fruit cup. Sprinkle with cinnamon and nuts. Garnish with mint leaves

Banana Smoothie

A quick and easy drink for those who aren't breakfast people.

Serves One

1 ripe banana	¼ teaspoon vanilla
¼ cup nonfat dry powdered milk	pinch of nutmeg
1 cup ice cubes	

1. Place all ingredients in blender until smooth.
2. Drink and enjoy.

Japanese Morning Delight

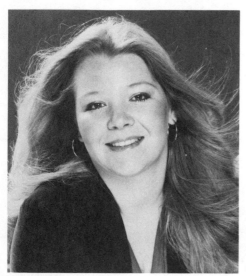

Name: Jeri Grubbs
Highest: 170
Now: 160
Goal: 120 to 115

I'm Jeri and I'm a good example of Yo-Yo Syndrome. I took off a whole lot of weight on Richard's Live-It and then I put it back on again. Now I've started on the Live-It again, after two months off, and I've already lost 10 pounds. I exercise 4 times a week in a class, and I'm real careful about what I eat. My mom is real thin, and she can eat anything, so she's a big help in the kitchen—she keeps inventing new things to try. Together we came up with this recipe—no, I'm not Japanese. But I did work for a Japanese bank once.

Ingredients

Serves Three to Four

3 eggs
1 cup bean sprouts, chopped
¼ cup chopped onion
2 tablespoons chopped green pepper

½ cup mushrooms, sliced
¼ teaspoon garlic powder
1 teaspoon tamari sauce

1. Beat eggs well and add remaining ingredients.
2. Drop egg mixture into hot nonstick skillet using a large spoon. Cook on both sides until golden brown.

Grapefruit Cups

A new way to zing up that old diet food.

Serves Six

3 small grapefruit
⅓ cup seedless green grapes
¼ cup unsweetened mandarin orange
    slices

1 small red apple, cored and diced
½ cup plain low-fat yogurt
2 tablespoons orange juice
    concentrate

1. Cut grapefruit in half. Cut around edges to remove grapefruit sections. Drain. Save shells.
2. Scallop edges of shells. Mix grapefruit with other fruits. Fill each shell with fruit mixture. Chill.
3. Before serving, combine yogurt and orange juice concentrate and top each cup with 1 tablespoon of this sauce.

From the kitchen of Renee Lognicon

Strawberry Egg Cakes

Let them eat egg cakes—especially these!

Serves Four

¾ cup creamed low-fat cottage cheese
¼ cup flour
⅓ cup nonfat dry powdered milk
¼ cup low-fat milk
½ teaspoon cinnamon or nutmeg

3 eggs, separated
1 cup strawberries, thinly sliced
1 cup strawberries, puréed
½ cup plain low-fat yogurt

1. Combine cottage cheese, flour, milks, and spice.
2. Add egg yolks and beat until smooth.
3. Beat egg whites until stiff peaks form. Gently fold egg whites into cottage cheese mixture.
4. Drop by spoonfuls onto a hot *lightly* greased nonstick skillet. Stud with sliced strawberries. Cook slowly so pancakes can cook through. Turn once.
5. Make strawberry sauce by combining puréed strawberries and yogurt. Serve pancakes immediately with the sauce.

Caribbean Cocktail

A refreshing drink that's really a meal.

Serves Two

2 bananas
1 cup fresh pineapple
2 cups milk

½ cup seltzer water
1 egg
1 teaspoon vanilla extract

1. Cut up banana and pineapple thoroughly.
2. Pour milk, banana, seltzer, and pineapple into blender. Blend at high speed until thick.
3. Add egg and vanilla and blend at high speed for two minutes. Pour into glass. Refrigerate remaining Caribbean Cocktail.

From the kitchen of Tracey Lord Lawrence

Live-It-Up Danish

At last a Danish to free you from coffee shop and packaged calories.

Serves One

2 tablespoons low-fat cottage cheese
1 tablespoon plain low-fat yogurt
¼ teaspoon vanilla or lemon extract

1 slice whole wheat bread, lightly toasted
¼ cup fresh peaches (or other fresh fruit), sliced
⅛ teaspoon cinnamon

1. Combine cottage cheese, yogurt, and extract. Mash together until fairly smooth.
2. Spread mixture on bread. Arrange fruit on top. Sprinkle with cinnamon.
3. Place in toaster oven or under broiler for 3 to 4 minutes until heated through, being careful not to burn.

Hurry-Up Fruit Shake

Shake it up baby, then you're on your way today.

Serves One

½ cup plain low-fat yogurt
½ ripe banana
¼ teaspoon lemon juice
¼ cup orange juice

1 cup fresh or frozen unsweetened fruit
⅛ teaspoon nutmeg

1. Combine all ingredients in blender until smooth.
2. Pour into chilled glass.
3. Drink up.

Yummy Breakfast Quiche

Quiche me you fool and allow 45 minutes to prepare.

Serves Four

8 ounces low-fat mozzarella cheese, grated
1 tablespoon Parmesan cheese
2 tomatoes, diced

1½ cups mushrooms, sliced
½ cup onion, diced
3 eggs
½ cup low-fat milk

1. Sprinkle half the cheese in bottom of glass pie pan or quiche pan.
2. Layer tomato, onion, mushroom, and remaining cheeses in pan.
3. Beat eggs and milk together and pour over top.
4. Place pan in a larger pan with 1 inch of hot water in it. Bake in 350°F oven for 45 minutes or until quiche is set all the way through.

Perfect Pancakes

Even Aunt Jemima would lose weight on these.

Serves Two

1 slice whole grain bread
1 egg
¼ cup buttermilk
2 teaspoons whole wheat flour
1 teaspoon baking powder

1 teaspoon honey
½ teaspoon vanilla
¼ teaspoon cinnamon
butter
¼ cup unsweetened applesauce

1. Blend all ingredients except butter and applesauce in blender or food processor until smooth.
2. Lightly butter a nonstick skillet. Make 3-inch (in diameter) pancakes by spooning or pouring mixture into hot skillet. Brown lightly on both sides.
3. Top with a dollop of applesauce.

From the kitchen of Marta Cerro

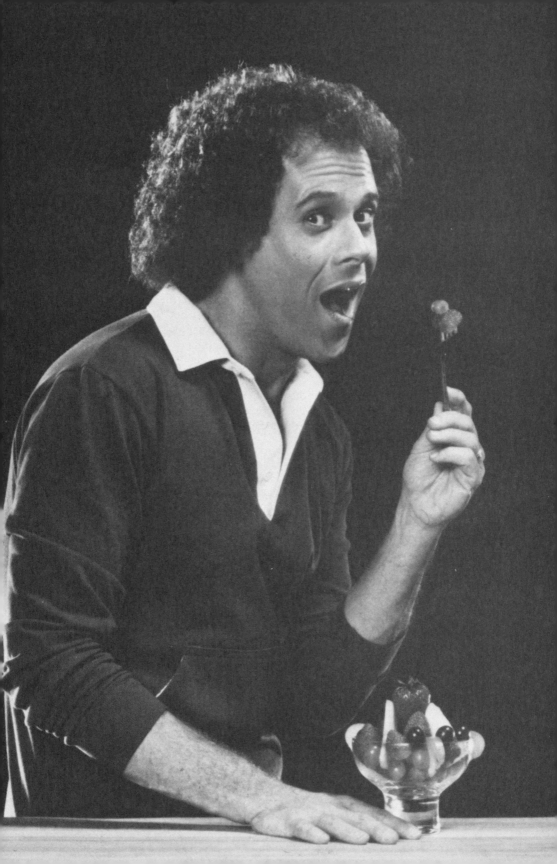

Time Out

BREAKING UP IS HARD TO DO

All right guys, here comes the bad news. That kaffeeklatch of yours has got to go. This is a raid. Kick Joe DiMaggio out of your home or office. Throw out those chocolate caramel donuts. Get rid of the Danish. I'm here to clean this place up and I won't take any hip from nobody. Got it?

Years and years you been in this here racket, drinkin' coffee, smoking cigarettes, eating gobbledygook till you bulge where you ain't supposed to bulge, causing your brain to go cock-a-doodle-doo from all that sugar and caffeine. I see it all, and sweetheart, this is the end of the line.

The junk stops here.

I'm cleaning up this town, and you are on my hit list. That means I'm going to come over and personally hit you if I see you put one more crumb to your mouth between breakfast and lunch. NO excuses, you get my drift? Snacks, coffee breaks, midmorning feasts—they're all going to end, now that I'm on the scene. They say that breaking up is hard to do, but baby, losing weight is even harder. So knock it off now, before the hips get any bigger.

There's plenty of things you can be doing with your spare time. You need a little pick-me-up. Well, pick up your rear end and march it around the building a few times. Take to the streets: Walk, run, trot, jog. Get off your duff and shake it up, honey. Twist and shout. Whether you work in an office building or at home, when you feel that need for a midmorning break—take it, but break with exercise, not food. Or you'll have me to answer to. Got it?

COFFEE, TEA, OR ME?

Many, many years ago, they did not have coffee. Adam and Eve drank apple cider. Alexander the Great drank wine. Nero drank grape juice. (He was A.A.) Then, one dark and stormy night, the Mufti of Aden was praying in the desert—which is where he happened to live. The Mufti was a very devoted man, but on this particular occasion, he found himself dozing off in the sand. Each time he awoke from one of these little camel naps (there were no cats in this part of the desert), he scolded himself and swore he would do better. The guilt was making him miserable. So the Prophet took pity on the Mufti and whispered in his ear the fact that when his goats ate the beans from a certain shrub, they would roam the sands mercilessly—awake the whole time, never drowsy, never sleepy.

The Mufti immediately took to munching on this same shrub and sure enough, he, too, found he was able to stay awake to complete his long and arduous prayers. But the neighbors happened to think he was nuts. A grown man eating a bush was a bit much for even them—and believe me, they thought they had seen it all. So the Mufti began picking the beans off the shrubs and cracking them between his teeth.

"There's got to be a better way," he used to say to his goats, to his wife, and to his children. (All of whom he regarded with mutual respect and admiration.) None of them could help him in any way. Then, quite by chance, there happened to be a great rainstorm in the desert. The heavens turned black, lightning crackled, and hot water burst forth from the heavens. You've heard of hail—rain so cold that it froze? This was rain so hot that it boiled. It all but flooded the Mufti's cache of coffee beans. But when it rains, it pours. And so the desert bloomed like the rose of Sharon, and the coffee industry was born.

The Mufti became a rich and famous coffee mogul—he soon bought a finca in Brazil and began writing songs for Frank Sinatra—and beans were no longer worth beans.

By the 1700s coffee was quite the vogue. By the 1900s millions of people were addicted to the warm rich brown liquid. Why was coffee becoming as popular as gold? Very simple. It contained caffeine, and we all now know that caffeine makes the heart go pitty-pat pitty-pat a little bit faster, which seems to perk up the whole system and give us a sense of refreshed vigor and renewed energy. So when the natural high goes dry, we just fill up with another cup of coffee.

And why shouldn't we? We watch TV and see our best friends drinking coffee. Mrs. Olsen is dispensing motherly advice and saving marriages with cups of coffee. Joe DiMaggio invites you to bring him home with you to brew some coffee. Even Marcus Welby says it's okay to drink a coffeelike drink. We dance to songs that sound like percolators at full speed. In no time at all some big fashion designer will come out with a designer coffee bean, I'm sure of it. People will stop trying to outsnob each other with their home grinders and their pounds of High Jamaican Blue and instead will make sure that only cream and sugar separate them from their Calvins.

Of course, a few people know the truth. And the truth is bitter. Caffeine is an addictive drug, and too much coffee is no good for you. So when you cut out your coffee breaks, do me a favor—cut out the coffee as well. If you want to drink something warm and soothing with one of your meals, try an herb tea. But take my word for it, you can get the same high you get from coffee with exercise, and you won't pay the price of damaging your body.

What? Are you kidding me? You've been sitting there reading this whole chapter with a cup of coffee in your hand? I don't believe you! Get up right now and throw it down the toilet. (And don't you ever drink coffee again while you're reading one of my books.) Now,

how about a little exercising instead?

Breathe deeply, and . . .

THE EXERCISE BREAK

Now that I've got you to dump out your coffee cup and stash your trash foods, I've got a new thing for you to try. C'mon, you've come this far with me, you might as well trust me a little bit more.

It's called the exercise break. It replaces the coffee break.

Whether you work at home or in an office, there's an exercise that you can do that won't mess up your dress-for-success navy blue suit or your brand-new Swirl housecoat. You don't have to take off your clothes; put on a leotard; and sweat, shower, and change. There are exercises that will just rev up your circulation and give you that good feeling that coffee or cola gives you, but they're better for you than anything you can drink.

I don't need to tell you that, of course.

Now, there's just one other point I have to make about midmorning (or midafternoon, for that matter) exercise. This is not a substitute for strenuous exercise. This is not the kind of exercise you do and then tell your friends what a hearty workout you've had or that you exercise religiously twice a day and couldn't live without it.

Exercise breaks are to replace coffee breaks—they get you away from your routine, they refresh your body and mind, and they make you think better. And that's not bad for fifteen minutes of your time, now, is it?

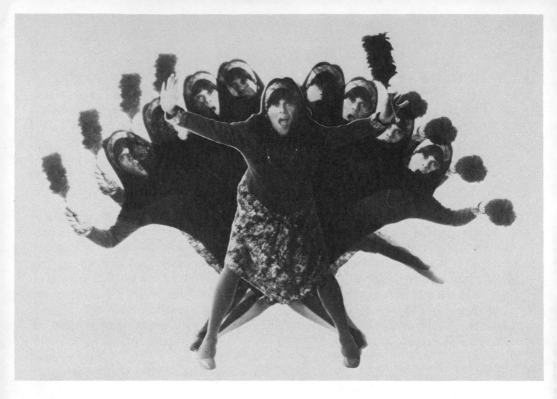

FOR PEOPLE WHO WORK AT HOME

Well, well, well. How did it get to be ten o'clock so fast? The morning just zooshed away with the speed of summer lightning and here you are, huffing and puffing from exhaustion, realizing that lunch is around the corner, and you still haven't even decided what to fix for dinner. The day and its tasks loom in front of you bigger than life. If you don't sit down for a cup of coffee, a little snack, and perhaps some television to help relax you, you just might freak out.

So you reach into the refrigerator for a little comfort. Perhaps you find the last piece of Pineapple Upside Right Cake. You might as well eat it because when the kids come home from school, they're just going to fight over who gets it. May-

be there's nothing sweet in the icebox, but there're two stuffed potato skins from the other night's dinner out. They're not enough for lunch, so you can heat them up for a midmorning snack. On second thought, as you begin to sniff them, maybe you'll just eat them cold. They really are so good, why wait five minutes and then risk burning your fingers? Maybe you're the Supermom type, so you've filled the ceramic cookie jar with home-baked oatmeal raisin-and-pecan snaps, fresh and crunchy for the kids' after-school snacks. The cake needs a cup of coffee or two to wash it down. The potato skins call for a cola. And only a glass of cold milk will make the experience of eating those cookies as satisfying as it should be.

So here it is 10:07, and you've already consumed 500 calories. Now, I don't go in for calorie counting, you know that. But I'm trying to be very graphic here because you have just offended your body in a graphic manner. If your daily caloric intake is 1000 to 1500 calories, what business do you have eating 500 calories at a nonmeal?

Let's take a minute and find out why you're really eating. Just answer these few questions. And don't worry if you haven't got a pen handy. Pick up any of those crayons on the floor. They'll do just fine.

1. A coffee break in the morning gives me the chance to:
a. legitimately quit the housework for a while.
b. call my girl friend and find out what's new with her.
c. enjoy the baby's morning naptime and remember that I'm a person.

2. For my break I usually:
a. meet my neighbor and drink coffee and talk about our children's problems.
b. leaf through a women's magazine and wonder why my house doesn't look like the one pictured.
c. plop down on the sofa and watch some television for some needed escape.

3. On my break I like to:
a. get back to that fabulous romance I was reading.
b. knit. Sweaters are really "in" these days.
c. nap. Seems like I'm always tired.

4. The best snack to accompany my coffee is:
a. something homemade and still cooling from the oven.
b. a leftover that will help me clean out the fridge.
c. a little packaged goodie like a chocolate Ding Dong or something neat like that.

5. I take a coffee break because:
a. I deserve it.
b. I need a rest.
c. I'm hungry and can't wait till lunch for something to eat.

How to Score

There's something very tricky about this quiz that I forgot to mention. If you took it at all, you've already scored. And you failed. There are no right answers. In fact, there aren't any good reasons to be having a coffee break. You had a good breakfast, right? (If you didn't have a good breakfast, put this book down immediately and wait until tomorrow morning; then eat a good breakfast and proceed.) Now, let's go over the quiz again. With the Live-It answers.

1. A coffee break in the morning gives me the chance to:
break my routine with a little exercise that will rev up my circulation and stimulate my mind and body.
2. For my break I usually:
meet my neighbors and we exercise together, having a great time.
3. On my break I like to:
exercise.

4. **The best snack to accompany coffee is:** no snack at all. And stop drinking coffee while you're at it. It may give you a little instant shot of personal electricity, but exercise will give you a better high that will last longer and be better for your body.

5. **I take a coffee break because:** my body is conditioned to some kind of break, and I've never broken out of the habit.

Pretty grim, isn't it? The Live-It answers look a lot different than yours, don't they? Well, live and learn, or Live-It and learn, as I like to say. Now you know. If you insist on taking a break from your morning, that's fine. But let's not screw up your body and offend your food plan. If you have a large amount of weight to lose, midmorning is just the time for your serious exercise program. I'd like to see you organize your time so you have forty-five minutes of sweat-producing (oh, excuse me, perspiration-producing) exercise. That way you'll have stretching and light exercising in the morning and a hearty workout in the midmorning. And you'll see results that will leave you a lot more satisfied than a piece of pie.

EXERCISES AT HOME

Midmorning comes around, your friend Judith drops by with baby Ross, and you two decide to sit down over a cup of coffee and talk about all your friends. Little Ross gurgles and coos, and the two of you have no difficulty at all in going through half a jar of freeze-dried coffee and two dozen peanut butter cookies. ("I'll just die if I don't get that recipe," says Judith.) By the time Judith leaves you've:

a. wasted twenty minutes.
b. gained five pounds.
c. had enough coffee to give you the shakes for the rest of the day.

So the next time Judith comes over, give her one of the armbands in the back of the book, and recruit her in your neighborhood exercise-break team. Get out in the streets, go door to door, find everyone in the vicinity, and get them to exercise with you. It doesn't have to be big-deal exercising. You don't have to have special equipment or buy a trampoline or begin lifting weights. There's nothing to join, no dues to pay, and only a little energy to gain. But that's better for you than a few cups of coffee and some cheap gossip, don'tcha think?

THE WARM-UP

Deep Breathing
• Stand up straight, shoulders back, neck tall, and feet apart (remember always to check your posture before beginning any of these exercises).

• Inhale through the nose, then let all the air out slowly. You are expanding your lungs and getting your heart started—there's no better way of beginning your morning than with proper breathing habits.

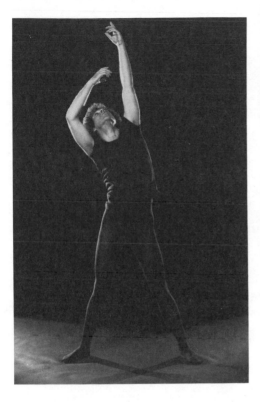

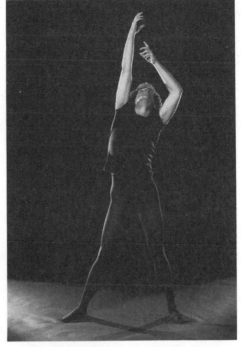

THE REAL THING

Many people who work at home see the size of their house as a huge problem: The bigger the house, the more they have to clean. They consider the stairs a private enemy and leave piles of items at each end of the staircase so they can be carried up or down by anyone who happens to be going up or down. Saving a trip up or down the stairs seems to be the main goal in their day. Not anymore! Get to those stairs and start marching. Walk up them and down, march up them with your knees coming as high to your chest as possible, jog up and down them, and then take them two at a time. This is great for your heart.

If you really can organize some friends, get an exercise class going in your living room or backyard. Better yet, make it the front yard—then everyone who drives by can see what you're doing.

Climb and Stretch

• Stay in your standing position, feet apart. Hold your stomach in, lift your neck high, and look at the ceiling.

• Bring both hands above the head as if you're ready to climb a rope. Alternate your breathing as you shift your upper torso. Right-hand reach as you *inhale*, left-hand reach as you *exhale*.

• You should feel all the pulling sensation in your shoulders and also from your waist (keep that stomach in, and tight).

• Just keep thinking about pulling that rope higher and higher. Come on, it's a rope, not a piece of dental floss.

For a midmorning class try these exercises:

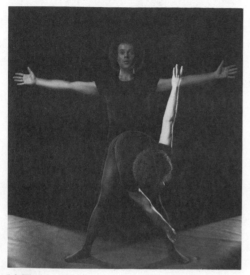 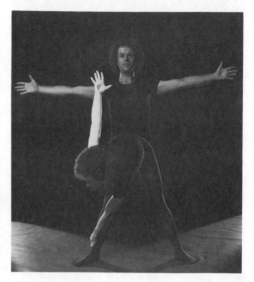

10 Toe to Toe

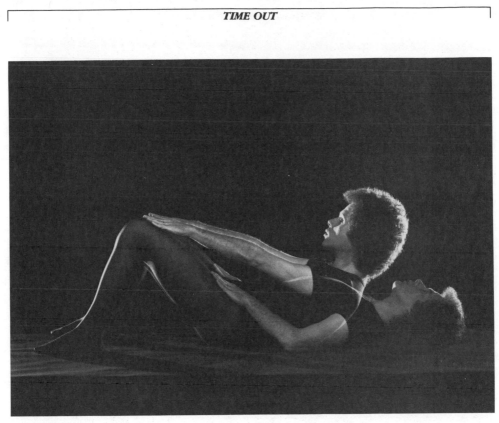

10 Mini Sit-ups

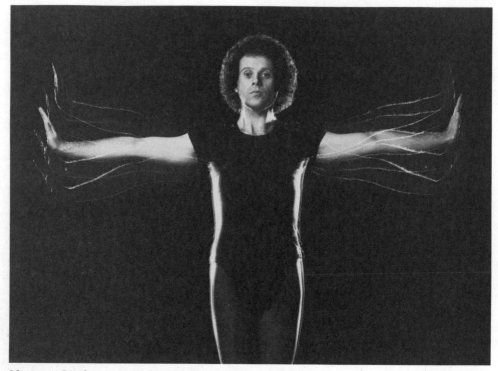

20 Arm Circles (10 each direction—no cheating)

20 Side Bends (10 each side)

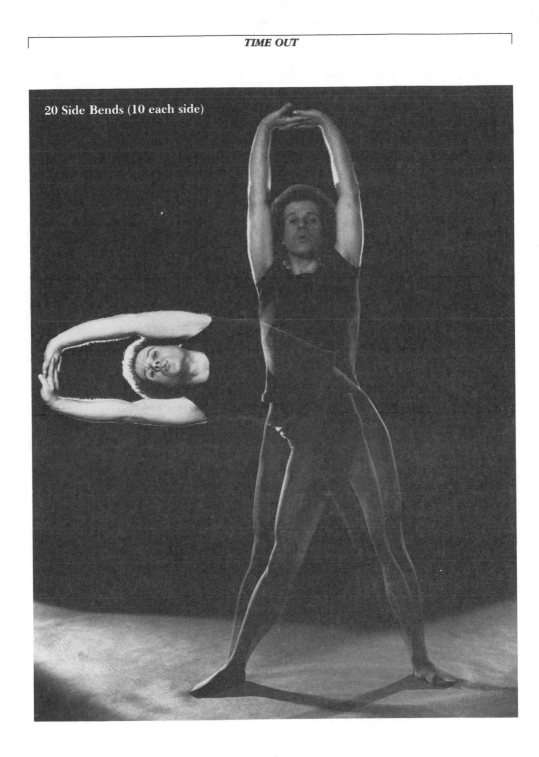

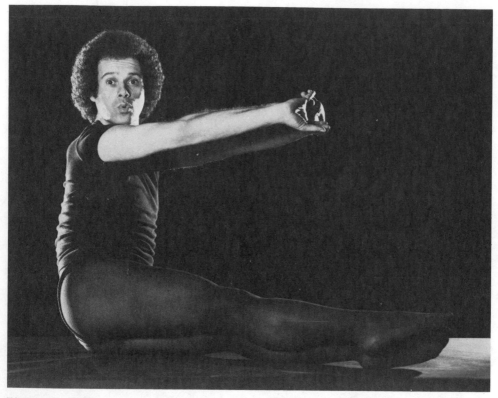

50 Tootsie Rolls

● Sit up straight, legs together tight, and extend your arms out again. Now all you have to do is lift up your rear one bun at a time and rock from side to side. ("Shall We Dance," from the musical *The King and I*, is perfect music.)

●Inhale while lifting the right bun, exhale while lifting the left bun. Remember to lock those legs and lift those buns as high as you can.

● As your thighs, hips, and rear are bouncing from side to side, make sure that stomach is held in. And where's your neck? Good, nice and high.

If you're going solo and don't want to do full exercises, get to those stairs, then walk around the block, then cool down with three very slow trips up and down the stairs.

There now. Don't you feel better?

FOR PEOPLE WHO WORK IN OFFICES

Well, you finally got your buns under that desk. It's about time. You could have been here twenty minutes ago if it weren't for all that dawdling you did between brushing your teeth and walking out the door. But I'm not the type to complain. I'll let bygones be bygones. I know you didn't stretch this morning. I know you didn't do your exercises. I know you skipped breakfast or drank a cup of coffee while you made the kids' lunches. I know that you're sitting there now, that you've been at that desk five minutes, and you've already got a headache.

You're bored. You're overworked. You have so much to do that you don't know where to start, and the day stretches on, impossibly long, without mercy or compassion. All you have to live for is your ten o'clock coffee break. In fact, your day is broken down into neat little packages, separated by breaks that make everything bearable.

By 9:15 you've had your first burst of energy, conquered the what-to-do-first crisis and are ready to glance down at your Timex to discover—hooray!—it's only forty-five minutes until you break.

By 9:30 you can stand it no longer. You

are pillaging through your desk drawers, wondering whatever happened to that half-started bag of Pepperidge Farm Milano cookies. Then you remember. You already ate them yesterday.

At 9:45 you've had another wonderful revelation: Lois brought in a homemade coffee cake this morning, so you won't have to eat those cardboard doughnuts from the coffee wagon. (No one forces you to eat them, but somehow you get them down in spite of their lack of taste.)

10:00: Two more minutes and you would have fainted from mere anticipation. A coffee break, you tell yourself, will give you that opportunity to wake up and tune in that you really haven't had yet. Your work will be better after your break, you're sure of it. And because you'll be working so much faster, you think you'll burn up whatever you eat midmorning—making the fattening food you are about to eat invisible to your waist, your hips, and your buttocks. Wrong. Even a one-calorie soft drink (with all those chemicals—yum yum yum) has to fit into your food plan. And the best mid-morning coffee break is the one in which you exercise your legs, not your jaws.

Go ahead, get up out of your desk and visit with your friends. But do it while walking up and down the stairs in your office building. If you ate a good breakfast (and you should have—it's the most important meal of the day, you know) then you should not be hungry by midmorning. If you're hungry then, it's for emotional reasons: You are bored, lonely, unhappy. You need something in your life. But it's not food. And it could be ex-

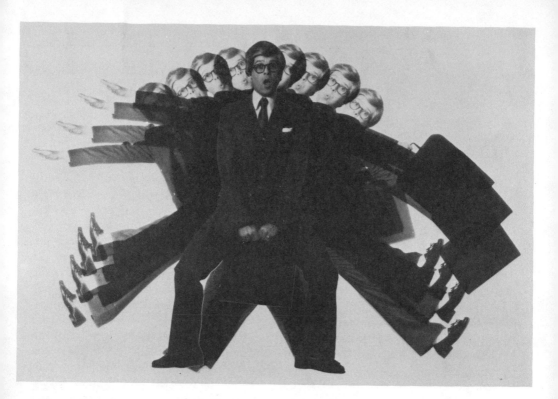

ercise. (It could also be a boyfriend, flowers from your husband, a raise, or a new dress.) But chances are, it's exercise. So step away from the stale atmosphere you've been stewing in and take a stretchercize break.

Organize an office exercise group. You needn't change into leotards, or sweat, or mess up your dress-for-success uniform. You do need to cut out the food. And the coffee.

EXERCISES FOR PEOPLE WHO WORK IN OFFICES

It's getting to be quite the fashionable thing to tell people who work behind desks that they should get out there and exercise. Health clubs offer business-

men's hours and special stenographic services so you can dictate to a secretary while you lift weights. Big conglomerates have gymnasiums right there in their office buildings. And cutesy-pie manufacturers invent all sorts of executive toys that are jokingly meant to encourage weight loss while still in shirt and tie, heels and suit.

I don't happen to believe in these gewgaws. Don't tell me you and your Rubik's Cube are getting a good workout. I've got other plans for you. So out from behind that desk. We'll do a little warming up—but nothing too strenuous, mind you. I don't want you to sweat or pull your shirt out of your trousers. It's so hard to get ahead in the business world when your clothes are rumpled and you've got body odor.

THE WARM-UP

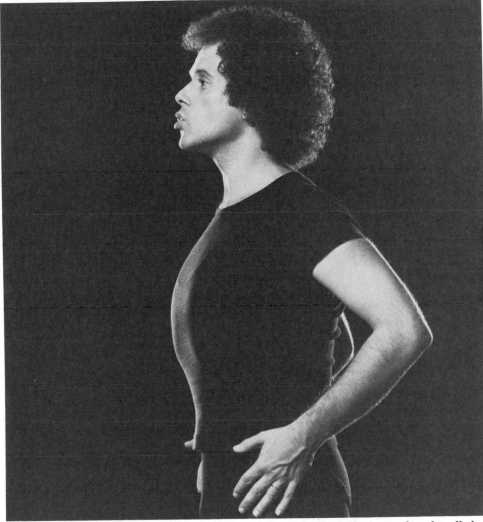

Deep Breathing

• Stand up straight, shoulders back, neck tall, and feet apart (remember always to check your posture before beginning any of these exercises).

• Inhale through the nose, then let all the air out slowly. You are expanding your lungs and getting your heart started—there's no better way of beginning your morning than with proper breathing habits.

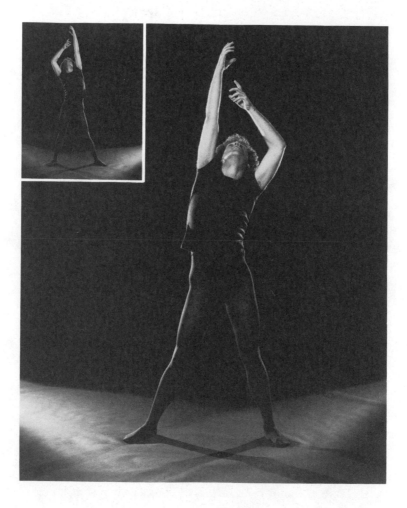

Climb and Stretch

• Stay in your standing position, feet apart. Hold your stomach in, lift your neck high, and look at the ceiling.

• Bring both hands above the head as if you're ready to climb a rope. Alternate your breathing as you shift your upper torso. Right-hand reach as you *inhale,* left-hand reach as you *exhale.*

• You should feel all the pulling sensation in your shoulders and also from your waist (keep that stomach in, and tight).

• Just keep thinking about pulling that rope higher and higher. Come on, it's a rope, not a piece of dental floss.

THE REAL THING

If you work in an office building, there's only one thing to do on your exercise break. Take to the stairs. Pretend the elevators are broken. Act out all the parts in *The Towering Inferno*. Get into the hallways and down the corridors and into those stairwells. The fire marshal insists that they be left unlocked, so don't give me any lame excuses. Start walking. Walk down and then walk up. Or walk up and then walk down. Go up the down staircase. I don't care, just do it. And while you're walking, pay attention to who else is walking.

Walking the stairwells is a great way to meet people.

Walking the stairwells is a great way to know whose job you can get next—if they're huffing and puffing before you are, they won't last long.

Walking the stairwells will help your heart, your lungs, and your leg muscles.

And don't forget to stand up tall while you're walking: Good posture is really important to your health—and your successful appearance.

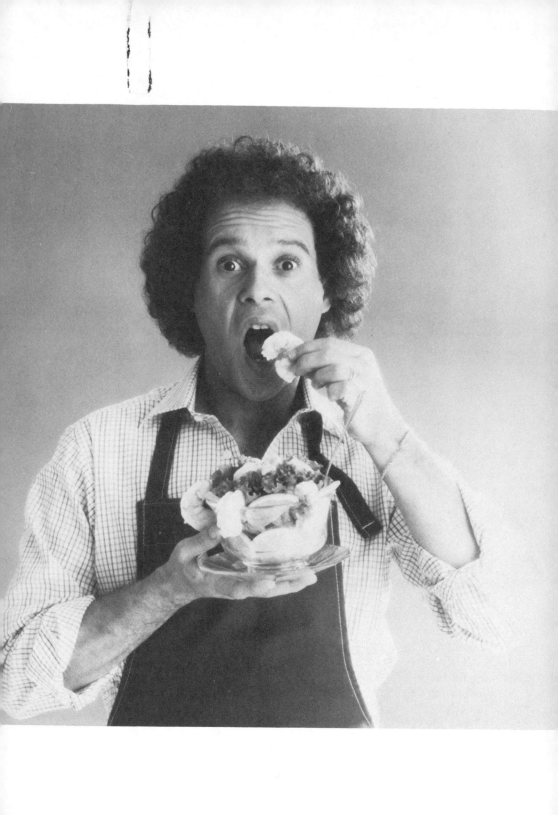

Lunge–I Mean, Lunch

ARE YOU THE LUNCH BELLE? TAKE THIS QUIZ AND SEE.

Up until now this has been a pretty easy book for you. It's been fun, it's been light, it's had some silly pictures—nothing that could tax the old brain too heavily. And every quiz I've given you has been kind enough to be multiple choice. I always liked multiple choice best when I was a student. You always knew one of the three answers was totally wacko, so you only had two to choose from and at least you had a fifty–fifty chance of getting it right.

No more. Now I'm going to get tough, because we're talking about lunch, and lunch is a very tough meal. This is a fill-in-the-blanks quiz. Now, don't be frightened and don't be scared. If you really care—and I know you do—you'll pick up your pen and get to work.

I'll give you a sample question so you can see how it works. SAMPLE: The meal that comes between breakfast and dinner is _____ .
See? That wasn't so bad, now was it? Now for the real test.

1. The meal that comes between breakfast and dinner is _____ .
2. The meal that gives us the most opportunity to experiment with foods is, _____ because after_____ you have several hours to work off the damage done by any fattening foods you have just eaten.
3. The sandwich is a perfect example of a food that was invented especially for _____ . Although usually made with two pieces of bread, for your _____ you should only eat sandwiches made with one piece of bread. And if you have bread with_____ , please don't eat bread again that day.
5. The meal you pack for your kids in a brown bag is _____ .
6. The meal you often take to the office with you is _____ .
7. A carton of yogurt, an apple, and a cup of coffee is a poor example of what many people consider a nutritious _____ . They are wrong.
8. When you go to a restaurant for _____ , you are often overwhelmed by the menu and end up ordering too much food—and eating it. You're actually worried that every business _____ you have to attend is turning out to be detrimental to your health. And you're right.
9. You always decide to clean out the refrigerator of leftovers just before you eat _____ .
10. Sometimes when you bring your_____ to the office you end up eating it for a mid-morning snack. Then you go out to _____ with your office chums and end up a little heavier than you should be.

Okay, that's it. Ten simple questions. How'd you like it? There's no fancy mathematics here because you don't have to score. Of course, you'd probably like to know what answers go in the blanks so you can see if you get a happy face on your paper, a gold star or a big red F. Well, it's all very simple. That's right, you sly dog you. The same word goes in all the blanks: Lunch! If you got 100% on this exam, you are certainly the Lunch Belle. There's a prize in the back of the book for you.

RICHARD SIMMONS' DOS AND DON'TS

Every time I'm on an airplane (which is an awful lot these days), I look at all the magazines they keep in the cubbyhole up front. The stewardess usually comes around and offers a magazine, but she only offers you one, because you have to share with everyone else on the plane. It's rude to say you want them all. But the truth is, I do. I want to read every magazine on the plane—the ones in the plastic

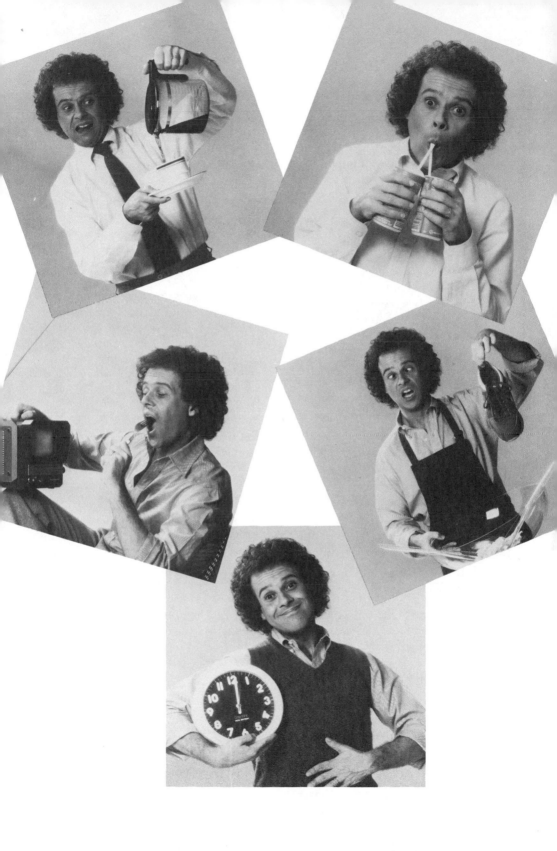

containers provided by the airline and the ones the passengers brought on board with them. I'm a magazine hog. And one of my favorite magazines is the one that has all these dos and don'ts in the front, like *Glamour*. The editors put a discreet black triangle over the person's face, so they won't embarrass him too much, but nonetheless, there they are, the doers and the don'ters of society. I always look for myself in the don'ts immediately. Then I sigh a little sigh of relief before I read the dos. The dos are never as much fun as the don'ts, but it's still my favorite section of the magazine.

I've made a list of my own lunchtime dos and don'ts. You can cut them out and save them. Or just turn to them every day when you look at your watch and get that joyous rush that means lunch.

DOS AND DON'TS

First the good news:
1. DO eat three well-balanced meals a day. No skipping, no skimping!
2. DO let the time of your breakfast and the amount of activity in your morning determine when you eat lunch. (High activity = four hours between meals; low activity = five hours; no activity = six hours.)
3. DO take a mental and physical reading of your being after eating lunch: if you're tired, drowsy, or in need of a nap—you ate the wrong lunch.
4. DO eat meals with company. Make your friends take the Lunch Pledge if necessary. (See p. 75 for Lunch Pledge.)

5. DO take exercise breaks rather than coffee breaks—get away from whatever you're doing to stretch and breathe and loosen up.

Now the bad news:
1. DON'T think you're hungry just because the clock says it's noon or six P.M.
2. DON'T duplicate foods. If you had eggs for breakfast, don't have egg salad for lunch.
3. DON'T have a soft drink more than once a week. (I'm a Pepper-Upper, too, but once a week and that's it. I know it's hard, but it's important.)
4. DON'T keep going through the kitchen on your way to errands—it's just too tempting to stop for a snack. Likewise DON'T cruise menus, meal trucks, or cafeterias looking at all the food before you decide what to eat. Make a selection before you enter—and stick to it.
5. DON'T eat any meals in front of the television set.

WHY? BECAUSE I LOVE YOU.

Why the DOS:
1. Every meal you eat should be a well-balanced one. It's just that simple. I, of all people, know that you are trying to lose weight. But your body needs proper nutrition, or it will fall apart. Your skin, your hair, your nails, and your mood—as well as your ability to perform even the simplest task—are affected by the foods you eat. Improper diet makes for an improper you. So eat right. Eat carefully. Avoid ding-dong food plans. Three small well-bal-

anced meals with no snacks in between and lots of exercise will get you the weight reduction you're dreaming of. I swear it.

2. You got up at ten A.M., you lazy bum. Don't tell me how you get away with that, but good for you. So it's ten o'clock in the morning before you even hit the shower. You do a few morning chores and before you know it, it's noon. At twelve ten you look at your watch and panic sets in. Oh, my word! It's time for lunch! Despite the fact that you got up at ten, ate breakfast at ten fifteen and haven't even had a chance to get hungry again, you are ready for lunch because the lunch bell in your head rings at noon, and you've been conditioned to believe that you must eat lunch between twelve and two. This is wrong. Wrong, wrong, wrong. If you ate the good breakfast you're supposed to be eating, there is no reason in this world you should be hungry in less than four hours. You can probably go five or six hours between meals, but you must go at least four.

We have all been conditioned, like Pavlov's dog (remember him from seventh-grade science?), to drool when we hear the lunch bell. There are two kinds of hunger—real true hunger and plain old appetite. Hunger means you must eat or die. Appetite means your mind tells you that you are hungry even though your body doesn't need any more fuel.

3. If you get that stuffed, heavy feeling after a meal—particularly lunch—you should not be drinking coffee to stay awake. You should be rethinking your menu. Lunch should be the happy break in the day that gets you out and away from your work and refreshes you for another round of work or pleasure. If you have no energy after lunch, you probably aren't on the right Live-It food plan. Or you've been cheating and aren't on a Live-It plan at all. It's better to leave the table a little bit hungry—and with energy—than to roll off the chair and curl up to a three-hour nap.

4. Eating with friends is one of the greatest social activities ever invented by mankind. But it can be very dangerous. Alone, you may eat a meager meal and be miserably lonely. But when your neighbor Pam comes over to see your wallpaper, and the two of you decide to lunch together, watch out, world—now you have a partner in crime, and lunch becomes a special occasion, so it's all right to forget about your food plan and feast on everything from leftovers to lasagna. So get smart. Eat meals with friends and have a good time. But make sure all your friends (and your family too) take the Pledge. And I don't mean Lemon Pledge.

On my honor, as a friend, I promise to stick to my personal food plan and to not bring any sweets, goodies, or sugary items into my friends' homes. Furthermore, I will eat, and allow my friends to eat, only sensible leftovers and healthful meals. I will expect my friend to stop me from eating anything that is not on my food plan and I will do the same for her. Together we will encourage each other to maintain or lose weight. I will not snoop in the Cookie Jar. I will not bring over magazines with pretty pictures of fattening foods. I will trust, love, and encourage my friend, now and forever. Amen.

5. Coffee breaks are the pits: You know that, I know that. And you can do something about them. Whether you're home or in the office, take an exercise break and get revived without artificial stimulants. (See Chapter 3 for some tips.)

Why the DON'TS:

1. Back to Pavlov's dog again. Don't let social conditioning ruin your waistline. Eat when you are hungry, not when you have an appetite. Or think you have an appetite.
2. The Live-It food plan is not one of those crazy diets that tells you what to eat on each day of the week. Basically you can have a little of any sensible food. So benefit from this variety. Don't eat the same foods. If you had bread at breakfast, no more bread that day. If you had a cola with lunch, no more cola that day. (Or that week!) Eggs? Just once, please. And watch the red meat. You will never get slim eating hamburgers.

3. Soft drinks have between six and nine teaspoons of sugar in them, and in case you haven't noticed, that's a heck of a lot of sugar. Low-calorie drinks have less sugar but more chemicals. Since the object of the meal is to help your body and not hurt it, I suggest you lay off the soft drinks. Try club soda or mineral water if you're dying for a little fizz. Try half a glass of club soda with half a glass of orange juice if you need a real pick-me-up.
4. Consider your kitchen enemy territory between mealtimes. Clean it and leave it. Don't keep walking through there to check out the cupboards, get the laundry detergent, or sniff out the electric burners. Put a combination lock on the door if you have to, but stay out. You can nibble yourself right into size 16½ without even sitting down to a meal.
5. I like television as much as the next person. Maybe more. But please remember that if your attention is on the tube and not on your plate, you may eat anything or everything that's in the house without even being aware of it. When it's time for lunch, take time out for yourself. Have a friend over. Or make things special just for you. Get away from your work. Get away from the TV or the book you're reading. (Even if it's this book—put it down.) Set yourself a special place at the table. Use real china and silverware. Don't eat out of containers. This should be a pleasant mental and physical break. Pay attention to the food and enjoy it. Then go back to whatever you were doing and feel refreshed.

ADVICE TO THE LUNCHLORN AT HOME

Almost any magazine you pick up these days has a big fancy spread in it about the new technology and how Americans are moving back into the home as their place of business. With computers and word processors and abracadabra machines, they are saving gas, saving lunch money, and saving time by staying at home. While this may be working for a few people—mainly the ones mentioned in the story—the people I meet fall into two different categories. There are people who go to an office or factory to work and people who stay home to work. The ones who stay home usually have a harder job—they have housework and children to look after and may not even have the opportunity to get out of the house or to mingle with surging crowds. It's for them that I give this advice to the lunchlorn.

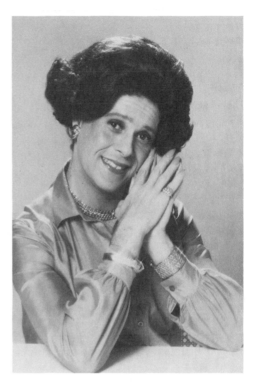

Dear Richard:

I am a twenty-seven-year-old woman with two young children. My day begins at six thirty in the morning and doesn't end until after eight P.M. when I put Greggy to sleep. (The baby goes to bed at seven.) Then my husband always wants me to rub his back and listen to his problems, and you know how all that goes. As a result I find I have no time to myself. I don't even have time to eat! During meals, I spend all my time cutting the kids' food or getting things for the table I forget to put there in the first place. Lunch is the worst because it seems to take three hours to prepare and serve. One meal for the baby, another for Greggy (he only eats Spaghetti Os), and then something for me. I end up having the shakes and stuffing anything I can into my mouth just to keep from fainting. And I usually have to eat standing up while holding the baby in one arm. Sitting down to three regular meals is a joke to me.

Love,
Joker's Wild

Dear Wild:

I get a lot of letters like yours and I am not unsympathetic. Raising children is one of the most difficult tasks there is—but also one of the most rewarding. Your life needs to be simplified so things have a little more flow to them and you don't have to run around so much. Why don't you get your husband to join you in the kitchen after you put Greggy to bed and have him help you prepare foods for the next day? You'll have time together to talk and you'll have the next day's meals under control before you go to sleep. You can wake up knowing that the day is going to be a little bit easier. And you'll eat more sensibly because you won't be grabbing at whatever junk food seems easiest to reach.

Love,

Richard

P.S. And send me a picture of the kids when you can—I'd love to see them.
P.P.S. Don't worry about Greggy's eating habits. When he gets a little older, he'll eat a more balanced meal. Just make sure you don't let him eat sweets.

Dear Dickie:

I have only one problem. I love to eat. My husband watches me really carefully and he's supportive of my weight reduction plans, but when he's out of the house, and I'm here alone, I slowly lose control. I take one cookie. Then I eat the bag of cookies. I plan on a salad for lunch—something healthful, you know—and then decide that the salad would taste better with a frozen pizza. Since I don't have frozen pizza in my house (my husband has inspection every week), I have to go to my neighbor's house. There we have pizza, salad, and cake. Afterward I feel real guilty. I'm also not losing any weight, and my husband is getting suspicious. What am I going to do?

Hungry for More

Dear Hungry:

What you should be hungry for is self-discipline. You're acting like a child, thinking that your husband can take care of you and tell you what to eat, when to eat it, and what you can keep in the freezer. You've got to realize that no one can lose weight for you but you. And until you decide to police yourself and take control of the situation, no one—not even me—can help you. I can talk to you till I'm old and shrunken, your neighbor can shop for you, and your husband can plead, but none of this will make a difference. The weight loss has to be your need and the discipline has to come from within you. Think about it for a while. Then if you want some help and support, let your husband, your neighbor and me, help out. But you've got to do most of the work yourself. And let me tell you, it's hard work.

Love,

Richard

Dear Mr. Simmons:

I love you and I think you're great and if you ever come to San Antonio I hope you'll give me a call (512) 555–0098, but I have so much trouble staying on a sensible food plan that I'm always in a mess. It's just too hard to go grocery shopping and come up with a master list of all the things I need for a week's family dinners, let alone special lunch meals for me. No one has that kind of time—or energy. I need quick and easy lunches. Cooking a big dinner is hard enough. Don't tie me to the kitchen any more than I need to be!

Tied and True

Dear Tied and True:

Just wait one second, my friend. You're getting all carried away. The Live-It is not one of those diets where you can only eat the prescribed foods in a fancy calendar that say things like *TUESDAY: half a breast of chicken, 4 carrots, 4 stalks of celery, and 1 tablespoon of fresh fruit.* The Live-It just says to eat light, sensible meals in small amounts three times a day. When you're shopping and cooking dinner, make an extra portion for your lunch the next day. Then all you have to do is warm it up. That's not too hard, is it? Don't start trying to create some new meal or start combining leftovers that will make your rear end look like the stern of the *Good Ship Lollipop.* Eating sensibly takes a little planning and that's it. So go to it.

Love,

Richard

Dear Dickie,

I am home all day by myself. It's wonderful to have some quiet while the kids are at school, and I like being alone long enough to get some housework done and then to enjoy the TV programs I like so much. But lunch is a very lonely proposition. Sometimes I invite one of my girl friends over, or the neighbor from across the street Marianne, but usually that's a disaster. I've discovered that two people convince each other to eat things they should not even be thinking about or have in the house at all. Now Marianne and I are hardly speaking, and I'm reluctant to invite any friends over. But I'm so lonely. What should I do?

Miserable

Dear Miserable,

I understand your problem. You seem to be damned if you do and damned if you don't. Well, don't go off and join a Miss Lonelyhearts Club, yet. There are several things you can do. You can turn Marianne into your lunchtime buddy and both take the pledge to help each other stay on your food plan. Or you can escape the house entirely during lunch. If you've been home all morning, there's no reason why you can't go out. Eat a light lunch by yourself and then go to the grocery store and have some fruit in the store. (Be sure to pay for it.) Or buy a cookie from the bakery in the mall and eat half of it. (Then walk the entire length of the mall twice to work it off.)

If you crave social contact (and who doesn't?) then get it. You needn't give up your Live-It. Just lay down the laws to your neighbors and friends.

Love,

Richard

Fish-filled Tomatoes

There's nothing fishy about these tomatoes—they're great!

Serves Six

6 large ripe tomatoes
2 cups cooked fish, flaked
1 cup cooked brown rice
¾ cup Swiss cheese, grated

1 egg
½ teaspoon oregano
1 tablespoon butter, melted
¼ cup whole grain dry bread crumbs
oil

1. Cut ½-inch slice from top of each tomato. Core, using melon baller, leaving ¼- to ½-inch-thick shell. Turn over and drain on paper towels.
2. Combine fish, rice, egg, cheese and oregano.
3. Fill tomatoes and place on lightly oiled baking dish.
4. Combine butter and bread crumbs. Sprinkle on top of each tomato. Bake in 350°F oven for 15 minutes.

Fruited Curry Luncheon Salad

If you like taste, have the good taste to try this one!

Serves Two

dash of allspice
dash of curry powder (to taste)
2 tablespoons mayonnaise
2 tablespoons plain low-fat yogurt
6 ounces cooked white meat turkey, cut into bite-size pieces

1 unpeeled red apple, cored and diced
1 orange, peeled, seeded, and diced
1 cup celery, sliced diagonally
¼ cup coarsely chopped walnuts
romaine lettuce leaves

1. Combine mayonnaise, yogurt, curry powder, and allspice.
2. Combine all other ingredients in large bowl. Pour dressing over, toss well. Chill.
3. Heap onto lettuce leaves.

Chicken Meatballs

Something special the colonel doesn't have.

Serves Two or Four*

½ pound cooked white chicken meat, ground
2 tablespoons green onions, chopped
¼ cup celery, diced small
¼ cup chicken broth

½ cup whole grain bread crumbs
½ cup tomatoes, chopped
¼ cup green pepper, chopped
½ teaspoon Vegit or Vegetable Powder

1. Combine all ingredients.
2. Form into eight balls and place on cookie sheet or pie pan.
3. Bake in 350°F oven for 30 minutes.

From the kitchen of Kris Cordon

*Makes eight meatballs. Serves two as a main dish. Serves four as a side dish.

Lettuce Burritos

Eat Mexican without gaining an ounce!

Serves Six

Lettuce leaves, large, dark, and flexible
1 cup fresh mint leaves, chopped
1 cup fresh parsley, chopped
½ cup fresh cilantro

1 cucumber, sliced thin
2 tomatoes, sliced thin
½ cup water chestnuts, sliced thin
½ cup red onion, chopped

Filling:

2 whole chicken breasts, skinned and deboned
1 cup water
½ cup red onion, chopped

1 tablespoon dill weed
½ teaspoon marjoram
Orange Vinaigrette or Poppy Seed Dressing (See p. 162.)

1. In medium saucepan, combine all filling ingredients. Bring to a boil. Reduce heat and simmer until chicken is tender. Remove chicken, reserve broth for soup or stock.
2. Shred chicken, place in serving bowl. Place all remaining ingredients in serving bowls. Place all bowls on table, buffet-style.
3. To make burritos, each person starts with 1 lettuce leaf. In center of leaf, add chicken and other ingredients of choice. Ladle dressing onto mixture. Roll up lettuce leaf like a burrito.

Quickie Quiche

A meal in a pie plate that you can still eat.

Serves Eight

1 tablespoon butter
2 cups broccoli florets or grated
   zucchini
1 cup leeks, sliced thinly
½ teaspoon dried dillweed, crushed
   pinch of salt
   pepper to taste
1 tablespoon tamari

1 teaspoon Worcestershire sauce
1½ cups skim milk
¾ cup nonfat dry powdered milk
5 eggs
¼ pound grated Swiss cheese
4 tablespoons freshly grated
   Parmesan cheese

1. Melt butter in skillet. Add broccoli or zucchini, leeks, and seasonings. Cover and cook over low heat 6 to 8 minutes; stirring constantly.
2. Beat eggs and milks together and set aside. Place the vegetables on bottom of 9-inch pie plate. Sprinkle cheeses over vegetables, reserving 1 tablespoon Parmesan cheese to sprinkle over top.
3. Gently pour egg mixture over all. Sprinkle remaining Parmesan cheese over top.
4. Place pie plate in shallow baking pan with 1 inch of water. Bake in 350°F oven for 50 to 60 minutes until toothpick inserted in center comes out clean.

Shrimp Cocktail

For special occasions—you eat this, don't drink it.

Serves Five to Six

1 pound shrimp, shelled and
   deveined
2 onion slices

1 bay leaf
1 tablespoon lime juice
⅛ teaspoon pepper

Cocktail Sauce:

¼ cup chopped onion
¼ cup diced celery
½ cup No Kidding Ketchup* and

½ cup tomato juice
¼ cup lime juice
   Worcestershire sauce to taste

1. Combine 2 cups water with onion slices, bay leaf, 1 tablespoon lime juice, and pepper. Bring to boil, drop in shrimp, reduce heat and simmer 3 to 4 minutes.
2. Chill in boiled water. Drain shrimp and reserve stock for soup.
3. Combine shrimp with Cocktail Sauce ingredients. Mix well and chill.

*See No Kidding Ketchup p. 161.

Stuffed Zucchini

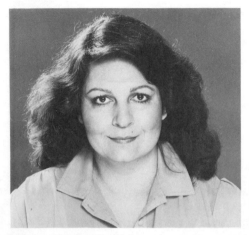

Name: Karen Warne
Highest: 275
Now: 249
Goal: 125

I'm Karen Warne, and the least I've ever weighed is 7 pounds 6 ounces. Since I was born I started gaining weight. I've been on every diet imaginable, but now I'm being good. I stick to the Live-It. No breads. Cheese is my big weakness. I also cut out salt. The other day I had Chinese food, and I was puffy the next day. I figured out it was the salt in the soy sauce. But I love vegetables and I experiment a lot. When I found out you could get a recipe in this book, I just worked on it until I got it right.

Ingredients

Serves Two

2 medium zucchini
¼ cup bell pepper, diced
½ cup celery, diced
½ cup onion, diced
1 clove garlic, minced
1 teaspoon butter
½ cup water chestnuts, thinly sliced

1 cup fresh mushrooms, thinly sliced
2 tomatoes (fresh or canned), finely chopped
3 ounces Jack cheese, shredded
⅛ teaspoon sweet basil
pepper to taste

Zucchini
1. Cut zucchini lengthwise and scoop out pulp, leaving a shell.
2. Steam for 6 to 10 minutes.

Stuffing:
1. Sauté bell pepper, celery, onion, and garlic in butter till tender-crisp. Add water chestnuts, mushrooms, and tomatoes and sauté for 2 more minutes.
2. Add sweet basil, pepper, and half the shredded cheese. Mix all ingredients and stuff the zucchini shells.
3. Bake in 350°F oven for 25 minutes.
4. Top with remaining cheese and place under broiler till cheese melts (about 1 minute).

Tabouleh-Stuffed Cucumbers

It's exotic but easy to make, and yummy in the tummy.

Serves Six

Cucumbers:

3 large cucumbers

mint sprigs for garnish

Tabouleh Stuffing:

¼ cup dry navy or white beans
1 cup chicken stock
4 cups boiling water
1¼ cups bulgur
¾ cup chopped scallions
1½ cups tomatoes, peeled and chopped
1½ cups chopped parsley
  pulp of 3 cucumbers

½ cup lemon juice
¼ cup red wine vinegar
½ teaspoon basil
¼ cup olive oil
¼ teaspoon black pepper
¼ cup finely chopped mint leaves
1 garlic clove, pressed

1. Score unpeeled cucumbers with a fork, and cut in half lengthwise. Scrape out seeds and pulp forming a hollow. Reserve pulp. Chill hollowed cucumbers.
2. Soak beans in water overnight. Drain. Add chicken stock, bring to boil, reduce heat and simmer for 1½ hours. Drain.
3. Pour boiling water over bulgur and let stand one hour until grain is light and fluffy. Drain and press out any excess liquid. Combine with beans.
4. Add all other stuffing ingredients, mix well.
5. Fill cucumber shells with tabouleh mixture. Chill. Garnish with mint.

Stuffed Bell Peppers
A new way to be a Pepper-Upper.

Serves Four

4 large bell peppers
1 tablespoon butter
1 carrot, grated
¼ head small cabbage, shredded
1 celery stalk, finely chopped
½ medium zucchini, grated

¼ cauliflower, chopped
½ medium onion, chopped
½ to 1 teaspoon oregano
1 clove garlic, mashed
1 tomato, chopped

1. Cut top (1 inch) off bell pepper and scoop out seeds and pulp. Steam bell peppers, and tops, for 5 minutes.
2. Melt butter in large nonstick skillet. Add remaining ingredients except tomato, and sauté until tender.
3. Add tomato and sauté 1 more minute. Stuff mixture into peppers. Replace tops. Bake in preheated 350°F oven for 30 minutes, until tender when pierced with a fork.

From the kitchen of Betty Wood

Tuna Imperial
It's the crowning glory of any table.

Serves Four

1 egg
¼ cup mayonnaise
⅛ teaspoon dry mustard
2 teaspoons Worcestershire sauce
1 tablespoon lemon juice
2 tablespoons plain low-fat yogurt
2 7½-ounce cans tuna, packed in
water

2 tablespoons chopped green pepper
2 slices whole wheat bread, cubed
¼ cup green onions, sliced thin
½ cup celery, chopped
¼ cup grated Cheddar cheese
lemon wedges

1. Preheat oven to 400°F. In medium bowl, combine egg, mayonnaise, yogurt, dry mustard, Worcestershire sauce and lemon juice. Mix well.
2. Drain tuna completely and add to egg mixture with the green pepper, green onions, celery, and bread cubes. Toss lightly with fork until well mixed.
3. Pour into 1-quart baking dish. Bake about ten minutes. Sprinkle top with cheese. Return to oven and bake five minutes longer or until cheese melts. Garnish with lemon wedges.

From the kitchen of Clara E. Davis

Chilly Cottage Cheese Mold

A light and refreshing way to enjoy cottage cheese.

Serves Four

1 package or 1 tablespoon unflavored gelatin
½ cup pineapple juice

2 cups low-fat cottage cheese
2 cups strawberries
salad greens

1. In small saucepan, sprinkle gelatin over pineapple juice. Let stand 2 minutes. Cook juice over low heat until gelatin is completely dissolved.
2. Combine juice, cottage cheese, and strawberries in blender or food processor until smooth.
3. Turn into a 1-quart mold. Chill until firm. Unmold onto salad greens. May garnish with a few fresh strawberries and mint leaves.
4. To serve, cut 2-inch slices and place on a bed of salad greens.

KIDS' LUNCHES

When I went to school, there were two different kinds of kids in the school. Those who brought their lunches and those who ate the school lunch. There were a few who did both—but they were athletes, and believe me, when you go to Cor-Jesu High, there aren't too many true athletes. The kids who bought their lunches all sat together on one side of the cafeteria, and the kids who ate on trays all sat at the other end. This wasn't a school rule or anything, it just seemed to be a chosen type of segregation that was never discussed in *Brown* v. *The Board of Education.* These two groups were very cliquey among themselves and each thought the other was more élite.

But I didn't belong to either group. I was the chubby kid who made all the jokes to get people to like me and I had a problem no one else seemed to have. I both brought my lunch and ate a school lunch but was not an athlete. That's because I always ate the lunch I brought before lunchtime and then, as soon as the bell rang after third period, I ran and got in line in the cafeteria for a hot lunch. If you got in line fast enough, you could get a lunch, eat it, and get in line again for another lunch just as the line was becoming a manageable length. And since I was a bit embarrassed that someone might notice I'd been in line twice, I stared down at my feet and never looked up. Whatever they put on my tray, I ate.

I was looking at a news magazine recently, and it had a story about school lunches in it. There was this big photo-graph of all the trays being dumped after lunch; each child had eaten everything on his tray except the green beans. There were green beans in stack after stack of dishes, and it looked like these poor kids were very wasteful. It also reflected poorly on the school and its lunch program. Well, my school never had that problem. Whatever the other kids didn't eat, I ate. In my lunchbox (the one with Roy Rogers, Trigger, and Dale Evans) I kept a Thermos filled with béarnaise sauce. A little dab of béarnaise got me almost anywhere—and green beans, squash, cauliflower, and diced carrots were my friends.

Since I was in school there's been a tremendous brouhaha over the nutritious benefits (or lack of) in some kinds of breads, or the lack of proper nutrition in kids' lunches, and all kinds of new questions about what to give the kids. We all know that the kids that don't have Fritos in their lunches trade with the kids that do, and that the kids with apples always toss the apples and buy the chocolate cake with icing the school lunch is offering.

So what's a responsible parent to do? If you've got the time and the money, I think you should send your kid with his lunch. But you have to make that lunch so interesting that he won't want to trade it with another child. The food has to be good to eat, it has to be good for you, it has to look good, and it should crunch.

Crunching is very important to children. Crunching gives them comfort. That's why potato chips are so popular. But vegetables crunch too—and don't you forget it.

Here's a few tips that might make your child more interested in the lunch you send him off with—and more likely to eat it.

Put a personal note in lunch to your child every now and then. Don't do it every day or it won't be special. Just something like "I Love You" or "Have a Nice Day" or some sweet special words that are meaningful only to the two of you.

Even though they cost a little more money, buy some of the canned juices and other products you like to use that come in small sizes. They're cute, and kids like them. Freeze a can of apple juice and then add it to the lunchbox in the morning. It will keep lunch cool during the morning and be thawed out by the time lunch comes around.

Investigate soft lunch bags, as well as the traditional lunchboxes. There seems to be a revolution going on in design, and now there are dozens of lunch carriers available. A different lunchbag every now and then might make the contents seem more interesting. Presentation adds a lot to flavor, and don't you forget it. Even for kids. You can make inexpensive and fun lunch bags from pillowcases. Choose a *Star Wars* or Snoopy or print pillowcase your child likes and sew it into a pouch that measures about 8 by 11 inches. Add drawstring and *voilà:* a lightweight lunchbag that can be stuffed in the jeans pocket after lunch rather than forgotten or lost along the way.

Tupperware and the other plastic manufacturers make cute little colored containers. Put foods in these and watch your child's delight. Colored utensils too!

Make sure the meal has a little of everything in it: Nutrition is the main idea, you know. But make sure there's something zingy there too.

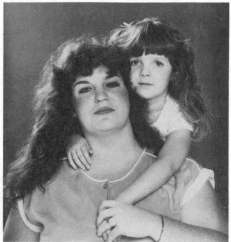

Name: Samantha Cederquist
Highest: 315
Now: 185
Goal: 125

My name's Samantha, but you can call me Sam. I've never had a weight problem until I became pregnant with my little girl, Larissa, that was in 1976. By the time she was born in 1977, I must have gained 80 pounds. When I was pregnant, I thought I had to eat for 4, to make sure she got the right nutrients. Then I was nursing and I thought I had to eat for 3. And I just never took any weight off, in fact, I gained even more. In February 1980 I read an article about Richard and I mentioned it to my dad. By coincidence my dad had done some lighting work at the Anatomy Asylum and he told me, "I've seen a lot of fat girls go in there." So I decided to try it. Everything Richard said was already in my head; it's just that suddenly it clicked. Everything made sense for me, and it all came together. I also liked being part of a group. We were all in it, for better or for worse, and we helped each other. In May 1981 I started working for Richard and helping other people who were overweight. I work out every day, seven days a week, and I eat even less than the Live-It calls for. I'm real careful about intake, especially now that I've lost so much weight. I eat two small meals a day and one medium-sized. And I'm real careful with what my daughter eats. I don't want her to gain on school lunches, so I send her to preschool with her own lunch.

❧ ❧

Apple-Blossom Sandwich
Celery Sticks Lightly Spread with
Peanut Butter
Milk

❧ ❧

Apple-Blossom Sandwich

Serves Two

2 slices whole wheat bread
⅓ cup Neufchâtel cheese
1 large red apple

2 scant tablespoons raisins or chopped
nuts
cinnamon

1. Lightly toast bread. Spread half the cheese on each piece of toast.
2. Cut apple into very thin wedges. Design a pinwheel with the apple wedges, pressing them lightly into the cheese.
3. Place raisins or nuts in the center of the pinwheel. Sprinkle with cinnamon. Wrap in foil.

Egg McSandwich
Fruity Shake
Carrot Sticks

Egg McSandwich

Have an egg McSandwich with McSimmons

Serves Two

4 slices whole grain bread or 1 whole
pita bread, cut in half
2 eggs, hard-boiled
1 tablespoon mayonnaise

1 tablespoon plain low-fat yogurt
1 tablespoon each: chopped celery,
grated carrot, green onion, and
chopped tomato.

1. Mash eggs, add all ingredients, and mix well.
2. Spread on bread or stuff in pita bread. Wrap in airtight plastic bag.

Fruity Shake

1 large ripe banana
1¼ cups fresh strawberries (or any
other fresh fruit)

2 tablespoons nonfat dry powdered
milk
½ teaspoon vanilla or strawberry
extract

Place all ingredients in blender. Whirl until smooth. Pour into plastic Thermos and store in refrigerator overnight, until ready to pack up for lunch.

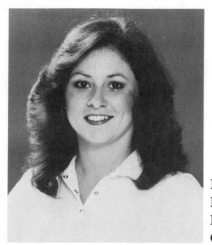

Name: Betty Zuniga
Highest: 228
Now: 138
Goal: 120

I'm Betty, and I work for Richard Simmons at the Anatomy Asylum. I've been heavy all my life. When I was ten, I was a chubby kid. In junior high school I was pudgy. I come from this Italian come-on-honey-eat family. I have no deep-seated psychological problems, I just eat because I was always told to eat. Then I got my weight down. After high school I weighed 128 and I was fine until I had a child when I was 22. I gained 60 pounds during my pregnancy, then I lost some, but then I gained about 80 pounds over the next 5 or 6 years.

Two years ago, through a friend, I met Richard—he greeted me at the door with open arms, and I felt welcome. On the first day I swore I wouldn't go back. But I did go back anyway. Richard just seemed to care so much. At first I didn't want to hurt his feelings. Then the dramatic results made me come back for myself. In the first month I lost 20 pounds. Now I'm Program Director for the overweight classes at the Anatomy Asylum. I'm on the Live-It and I exercise at least four times a week. My daughter, Kristina, is seven and next fall she'll be in the third grade. Every day I pack her a lunch so she doesn't have to eat in the school cafeteria. You have to watch what you eat at an early age, or you can be very unhappy.

🦎 🦎

Not-So-Chilly Chili
1 Piece Fresh Fruit

🦎 🦎

Not-So-Chilly Chili

Serves Six

1 tablespoon olive oil	1 bay leaf
½ cup onion, minced	¼ teaspoon oregano
1 clove garlic, minced	1 teaspoon cumin
1 cup tomato sauce	1 teaspoon basil
1 pound Italian tomatoes, chopped	white pepper to taste
1 large celery stalk, diced	2½ cups kidney beans, cooked
1 to 2 tablespoons chili powder	

1. Heat oil in large saucepan. Sauté onion and garlic until onions become translucent.
2. Add all remaining ingredients except beans and bring to a boil. Reduce heat and simmer 20 minutes. Adjust seasonings.
3. Add beans and let simmer 10 to 15 minutes more.
4. To serve for child's lunch, reheat and immediately place in insulated Thermos.

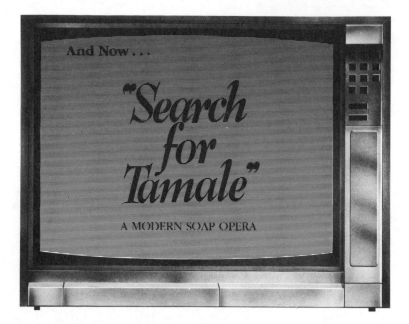

Music up: Da dum, da dum, dee dee da dum, dum te dum, la la, de tum, ta ta.

Scene One: The kitchen at Maura's house. You know the kitchen: the one with the white linoleum floor, the white Formica with the silver specks in it, and the new yellow and orange wallpaper in the old-fashioned quilt pattern Maura learned how to hang herself after the two-for-one sale at Wallpapers to Go.

A Panasonic coffeemaker brews in the background. A Gelatio ice-cream maker whirs. The house smells of coffee and strudel. The digital clock on the Amana microwave oven beats electric green: 11:37.

Enter Felicity. Maura's neighbor and best friend.

MAURA: Why, Felicity! How nice to see you. I was just doing the breakfast dishes. Want a cup of coffee?

FELICITY: Yeah, and make it a double. And have you got any rum to put in it?

MAURA: Rum in your coffee at this hour? It's only 11:38. (PAN TO SAME DIGITAL CLOCK ON THE MICROWAVE. ONE MINUTE HAS PASSED SINCE THE DRAMA BEGAN. HOW TIME FLIES WHEN YOU'RE HAVING FUN.) And you don't even drink wine! What's happened?

FELICITY: Happened? Nothing's happened. Nothing at all. What makes you think there's a problem? (SHE PICKS UP HALF–EATEN SLICE OF FRENCH TOAST AND BEGINS EATING IT, MOPPING UP MAPLE SYRUP WITH HER FINGERTIPS.) What would even make you ask?

MAURA: Felicity! We were roommates in college. You've been my best friend since we were eight. I dated your husband. I was matron of honor at your wedding. I held your hand the day after you got raped. I was at your bedside when you had meningitis. I brought you flowers when you had a miscarriage. I'm your daughter's godmother. You're *my* daughter's godmother. I think I know you pretty well, Felicity. I'd say we've been through a few things together. So whatever's bothering you—and I know something is (CAMERA PANS TO FELICITY, WHO IS NOW MOVING THROUGH THE TOP SHELF OF THE REFRIGERATOR, EMPTYING TUPPERWARE CONTAINERS AND EATING LEFTOVERS)—you can tell me all about it.

FELICITY: (BURSTING INTO TEARS) It's—it's—it's—it's—Scott. We're having problems. (SHE BLOWS HER NOSE IN A FLOWER–PRINTED BOUNTY PAPER TOWEL AND CONTINUES TO PROWL THROUGH THE FRIDGE.)

MAURA: Financial problems? You know Kevin and I would be glad to help out.

FELICITY: No, no. (SHE EATS HALF A COLD PIZZA WITH SAUSAGE AND MEATBALLS AND A LEFTOVER CAN OF BLACK OLIVES.) It's not money. You know Scott sold that piece of land his father left him. We're fine financially. It's per-per-personal.

MAURA: How personal? (SHE DUMPS THE OLIVE JUICE DOWN THE SINK.) He doesn't beat you, does he? I'll kill that bastard if he ever lays a hand on you. Why I remember once when he tried to . . . (MAURA BLUSHES) Oops. C'mon Felicity. I just cleaned the freezer yesterday. There's nothing there except for some French-style greenbeans and half a container of home-made lemon sherbert. Is it Krystal? Is she having a problem in school? Tell me, darling, tell me. You'll feel so much better.

FELICITY: (MOVING FROM FREEZER COMPARTMENT TO TRASH COMPACTOR, PICKING OUT BITS OF TOAST TO SCRAPE EGG BITS OFF THE PLATES STILL STACKED IN THE KITCHEN): No, Scott could never hurt me. And Krystal's just fine. It's w-w-w-worse than that, Maura. (SHE BURSTS INTO TEARS AND DISSOLVES IN HER FRIEND'S ARMS, SOBBING AND BLOWING HER NOSE IN MAURA'S APRON.)

MAURA: There there, Felicity. Now, don't fret. Everyone has some kind of sexual problem now and then. They're not really problems, my dear. Don't even look at it that way. It's not anything kinky, is it?

FELICITY: Kinky? Are you crazy? I'm not talking about a sexual problem. I'm talking about an addiction. I can't get Luke out of my mind or off my television set. What can I do?

MAURA: Well, I know exactly what to do. Let's treat ourselves to something really special. That'll make you feel better. Let's get dressed and go and buy *Richard Simmons' Never-Say-Diet Cookbook*. I hear he's got some great, low-cal recipes to eat while watching the soaps.

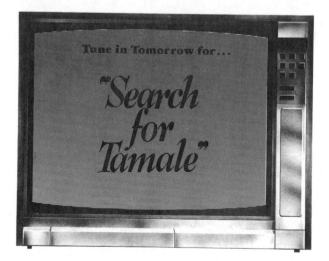

All My Children's Lunches

Make these so the kids don't bother you during your favorite lunch-time soaps.

Serves One Each

Pick-a-Pita Lunch

Cut pita in half, open, and fill with any of the following:

A. sliced turkey or chicken
sliced tomato
sliced cucumber
2 thin slices cheese
mustard to taste

B. 1 package falafel mix
sliced onions
sliced tomatoes
1 cup cucumber, sliced
½ cup yogurt
1 tablespoon fresh lemon juice
oil

C. flaked tuna, packed in water
sliced mushrooms
chopped scallions
Orange Vinaigrette dressing (See p. 162).

1. Prepare falafel according to package directions but *do not fry in oil*! After falafel is rolled into balls, place on lightly oiled baking sheet and bake 25 minutes at 375°F.
2. Place yogurt, cucumber, and lemon juice in blender, and process until smooth.
3. Put 3 falafel balls, onion, and tomato into pita bread. Spoon 2 to 3 tablespoons cucumber mixture over.

Banana Burrito

Serves One Each

1. Spread a tortilla, crepe, or chapati lightly with peanut butter.
2. Peel a banana and place at edge of tortilla. Sprinkle with cinnamon.
3. Roll up like a burrito. Wrap in foil if it's a brown bag lunch.

Apple Surprise

Cut 1 apple in half. Core. Spread inside with peanut butter, push apple halves together. What an unexpected treat!

The Young and the Ratatouille
A great tasting lunch without meat.

Serves Six to Eight

3–4 tablespoons oil
  2 large onions, chopped
  2 cloves garlic, minced
  1 medium eggplant, chopped
  6 medium zucchini, chopped
  2 bell peppers (red or green), cut in
    small thin slices

1 teaspoon basil
½ teaspoon thyme
½ cup parsley
4 large tomatoes
1 cup grated Jack cheese

1. Heat oil in large skillet. Cook onions and garlic until glazed. Add eggplant, zucchini, bell peppers, and spices. Cook until eggplant is almost done.
2. Add tomatoes and cook 15 minutes. Sprinkle cheese on top.
3. Cover and let cheese melt, or put in casserole dish, cover with cheese and bake in 350°F oven until cheese melts.

Days of Our Liver Pâté
Grandma called it French chopped liver.

Serves Four*

1 tablespoon butter
4 green onions, chopped
½ pound chicken livers
1 tablespoon white vinegar
½ teaspoon garlic salt or ¼ teaspoon
  garlic powder

3 tablespoons ricotta cheese
2 tablespoons fresh parsley
1 egg, hard-boiled
3 tablespoons dry white wine

1. Sauté onions in butter until glazed. Add liver and sauté until cooked thoroughly and brown.
2. Add vinegar and garlic, cover, and simmer 5 minutes. Let cool.
3. In blender, purée liver with egg, wine, ricotta, and parsley. Chill.
Serve with sliced raw vegetables (carrot sticks, jicama, celery, zucchini).

*As an appetizer. Serves two as a main course.

Guiding Bite Finger Foods
Light up your life with these treats.

Serves Four to Six

Pickled Crackers
12 whole wheat crackers
12 slices dill pickle

12 thin 1-inch square slices of Cheddar
  cheese
garlic powder

1. Place 1 pickle on each cracker. Top with a cheese slice and sprinkle with garlic powder.
2. Run under broiler until cheese melts.

Zany Zucchini

Serves Two to Four

4 ounces Neufchâtel cheese
2 tablespoons parsley
½ teaspoon garlic powder

1 tablespoon pimiento
1 medium zucchini, sliced lengthwise

1. Place cheese, parsley, garlic powder, and pimientos in blender. Mix until smooth.
2. Spread thin layer of mixture onto each zucchini half. Slice zucchini into 2- to 3-inch pieces.

Stuffed Mushrooms

Serves Six to Eight

16 large mushrooms
2 tablespoons butter
½ pound zucchini, chopped
5 green onions, sliced

1 clove garlic, minced
½ teaspoon Italian seasoning
1 teaspoon Worcestershire sauce
¾ cup shredded cheese

1. Remove stems from mushrooms to create a small hollow in each cap. Slice stems.
2. Melt 1 tablespoon butter in large skillet. Sauté mushroom caps for 1 to 2 minutes, being careful not to break them. Remove.
3. Add remaining butter, zucchini, onions, garlic, seasoning, and reserved stems. Sauté for 3 to 5 minutes. Stuff mixture into mushroom caps. Top each with a little cheese. Run under broiler until cheese melts.

Search for Tomato
Vegetarians can stop searching!

Serves Four

4 medium tomatoes
1 cup mushrooms, chopped
1 tablespoon butter
1 cup zucchini, grated
¼ cup green onions, finely chopped
½ teaspoon turmeric

½ teaspoon celery seed
¼ teaspoon garlic powder
¼ teaspoon onion powder
1 cup cooked brown rice
¼ cup cooked wheatberries
¼ cup walnuts

1. Cut tops off tomatoes. Scoop out pulp, leaving ¼- to ½-inch shell. Turn over and drain on paper towels.
2. Heat butter in skillet. Sauté mushrooms, zucchini, and green onions. Add spices and simmer. Add rice, wheatberries, and walnuts. Toss.
3. Stuff tomatoes with mixture. Place in 350°F oven for 15 to 20 minutes.

Ryan's Hope-You-Like-It Almost Irish Stew

An Irish Stew that's a little bit different and that's no blarney.

Serves Four

5 chicken breasts, skinned and boned
2 tablespoons butter
2 tablespoons wheat flour
1 medium onion, quartered
1 stalk celery, chopped into large pieces
½ bell pepper, chopped into large pieces
2 medium zucchini, chopped into large pieces

4 carrots, chopped into large pieces
1 medium red potato (with skin), chopped into large pieces
¼ cup parsley
2 cups chicken broth
½ teaspoon basil or thyme
pepper

1. Cut chicken into bite-size pieces. Place in plastic bag with flour and shake. In soup kettle or large pot, lightly brown floured chicken in butter.
2. Add broth and all vegetables and seasonings. Simmer until carrots and potatoes are cooked (firm). If broth is too thin, add 1 tablespoon flour dissolved in a little water and cook a few more minutes.
3. Season with pepper.

Doctor's Dilemma: Open-Faced Sandwichettes

What to eat when you're feeling not-so-hot.

Serves Two*

2 tablespoons cottage cheese
½ teaspoon prepared mustard
½ teaspoon Parmesan cheese
  a few sprigs of watercress

2 slices whole wheat bread, toasted
1 tomato, sliced
1 tablespoon plain low-fat yogurt
¼ teaspoon basil

1. Mix together mustard, Parmesan, watercress, basil, yogurt and cottage cheese.
2. To toasted bread, add tomato slices and cheese mixture. Broil until melted.
3. To serve as appetizers, cut each piece of toast in 4 pieces. Otherwise enjoy them as open-faced sandwiches.

*Or Four as an appetizer.

One Loaf to Live

A delicious stuffed turkey loaf.

Serves Six to Eight

Loaf:

2 pounds fresh ground turkey
2 eggs, beaten
½ cup buttermilk
1½ cups whole grain or sourdough
  bread crumbs

½ teaspoon Tabasco (less, if you're not
  a chili fan)
½ teaspoon oregano
½ teaspoon Italian seasoning
1 cup fresh tomatoes, peeled and
  chopped

Stuffing:

1 small zucchini, sliced
1 carrot, sliced

4 thin slices mozzarella cheese
¼ teaspoon dried basil

1. Combine all Loaf ingredients. Place half in lightly oiled loaf pan.
2. Steam zucchini and carrot for 5 minutes. Make a well down the center of the mixture in loaf pan. Layer zucchini, carrot, cheese, and basil in well.
3. Place remaining loaf mixture on top. Mold into a loaf, being sure to seal edges so cheese remains inside.
4. Bake in a preheated 350°F oven for about 1 hour.
   Great as a cold leftover.

As the World Turnovers

A fruity dessert for special occasions.

Serves Eight or One Turnover Each

Dough:

2¼ cups whole wheat pastry flour
1 tablespoon baking powder
½ teaspoon baking soda
4 tablespoons nonfat dry powdered milk
½ teaspoon allspice

dash of salt
½ cup vegetable oil
2 tablespoons honey
⅔ cup milk

1. Mix dry ingredients in a large bowl. In separate bowl, mix together wet ingredients. Make a well in center of dry ingredients. Pour in wet ingredients and mix well. Add more flour if necessary to form a stiff dough.
2. Lightly oil your hands and shape dough into a roll with a 2½-inch diameter. Wrap in wax paper and foil and refrigerate for a few hours or overnight.
3. Cut off 1-inch slices, and roll into 6-inch circles. Add 1 to 2 tablespoons fruit mixture, fold in half, pinch ends together. Bake in 400°F oven until golden brown.

Filling:

¾ fresh fruit juice (pineapple or apple)
1 tablespoon and 2 teaspoons arrowroot

1 cup fresh fruit (peaches, plums, or strawberries)
2 teaspoons cinnamon

1. Heat juice with arrowroot until thickened.
2. Slice or dice fruit and add to juice. Season with cinnamon.
3. Simmer until fruit is very soft. Let cool slightly.

Or try this variation.

Filo-Dough Apple Turnover

Serves Two

1 large apple, cored and diced
2 teaspoons lemon juice
1 tablespoon raisins, soaked in water
cinnamon
nutmeg

4 teaspoons plain low-fat yogurt
2 sheets filo dough
1½ teaspoons butter
2 teaspoons honey
2 teaspoons finely chopped nuts

1. Put lemon juice and ½ teaspoon butter in a nonstick skillet. Add apple, cinnamon, and nutmeg and sauté until apple is softened. Stir in raisins and yogurt.
2. Fold each sheet filo dough into a small square of about 5 inches. Place apple in half of filo dough square. Fold diagonally to form a triangle.
3. Seal and brush tops with glaze made of 1 teaspoon melted butter, honey, cinnamon, and nutmeg; sprinkle with nuts.
4. Place turnovers on lightly greased baking sheet. Bake in 350°F oven until lightly browned.

General Hospitality Rx

Serve these to your chums when they come to watch the soaps.

A.
Mix ½ cup crushed pineapple into 1 cup Neufchâtel cheese. Use carrot sticks as dippers.

B.
Mix chili sauce (to taste) and ½ teaspoon garlic powder with 1 cup Neufchâtel cheese. Spread on dill pickle slices.

C.
Put slices of sharp Cheddar or Jack cheese on apple slices.

D.
Mix 1 cup low-fat cottage cheese, ¼ cup finely chopped green olives, 1 tablespoon mayonnaise, 2 to 3 tablespoons pimiento, and ¼ cup plain yogurt in a blender. Spread a thin layer on celery stalks. Cut stalks into 3-inch pieces. Chill and serve.

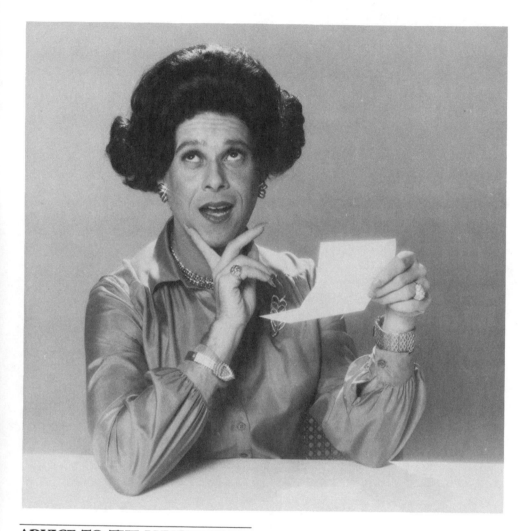

ADVICE TO THE LUNCHLORN AT THE OFFICE

People who work out of the home have an entirely different set of problems at lunchtime than people who work in the home. Yet, for both the lunch hour (or hours!) is fraught with pitfalls and opportunities to go astray. For those of you in offices lunch is a very social time of the day, and being around people often makes you eat more than you should. So knowing about the Lunchtime Traps before you fall into them will help you avoid them.

Trap #1
Dear Richard,

I have a terrible problem. I have just taken a job with a new firm. I love my job and think I will be very happy here. But it's in a new-business part of town, and every day the construction workers finish another high-rise office tower. As soon as the building is finished ten new restaurants open up on the lobby floor. Every day my friends want to try a new restaurant. I think I'll be twenty pounds heavier if I don't quit my job. What should I do?

Lobbyist

Dear Lobbyist,

Yours is a very common problem. Many people actually choose the jobs they will take by what restaurants are in the neighborhood. And wherever people congregate to work, restaurants continually spring up—be it near hospitals, factories or office buildings. While it's nice to get out of the office and enjoy a pleasant meal with your friends in a restaurant, it's no good for your figure if you sit down to a big meal and then have to sit at a desk for hours afterward without any way of exercising.

So here's a way out of your dilemma. On one of your lunch breaks or during a coffee break—if you have the time—make a survey of all the restaurants in your neighborhood. Ask to see the menus and write down the foods on the menu that are on your Live-It plan. Find the restaurant that will broil chicken or fish or serve a nice healthful salad. Avoid the restaurants that serve huge family-style meals with biscuits and potatoes and honey and beer and sour cream–based salad dressings. Once you know which places serve the kind of food you should be eating, stick to them. Then don't look at the menu when you arrive for lunch—just order from your mental list of acceptable foods. You'll have a nice time and still get a good meal—without gaining weight!

Love,

Richard

Trap #2
Dear Mr. Simmons:

I have a very erratic schedule. Sometimes I just have to stop and grab a bite to eat wherever I happen to be. I don't like to go into a big restaurant alone—they're expensive and time-consuming, besides the fact that I'd rather not eat alone. So I end up stopping at a fast-food restaurant for fried chicken, or a burger and fries, or a pizza. As a result, my skin is breaking out, and my hips are spreading. I'm very active, but exercise doesn't seem to control my weight.

Burger Buns

Dear Buns:

Junk food didn't get its name by accident. I'd like to see someone drive through one of those eatout/takeout places and have that little box you order talk back to them. Why doesn't the voice ever say, "Have you had a good salad today?"

A lot of people have your problem, Buns, and I'm sympathetic. Salesmen who are on the road know that time is money and they end up eating nonnutritious and fattening lunches from the kinds of places you describe. Women who run a lot of errands or who have small children often go to these restaurants as well. They're inexpensive and time-saving. I do know what you're talking about.

But I've got a way for you to avoid the trap. I think you're a perfect candidate for a bring-your-own lunch. Pack yourself a wonderful lunch in the morning and put it in an attractive basket, with a real fabric napkin. Then put it in your car. No Miss Piggy tin lunchbox for you. Make yourself what I call a European meal. Salad ingredients. A piece of French bread, or some crackers. A little piece of cheese. Some turkey slices. Keep the salad dressing in a little container so your salad doesn't get soggy.

When you're ready for lunch, stop at a park or a shopping mall. Set up your nice lunch and enjoy it. You'll be surrounded by people and a nice atmosphere and you'll have a nutritious meal that won't cost you too much. Then you can walk around the park or the mall and enjoy the sights and sounds before getting back in your car for more grueling miles.

Love,

Richard

Trap #3
Memo to: Richard Simmons
Dear Richard,

My problem is very simple. I work in a factory and there is only one place to eat lunch: the company cafeteria. The food is well priced and there's a big chart on the wall telling you how to compose a well-balanced meal, but I still find that I'm gaining weight. Cafeteria food should just be applied directly to my thighs! Should I be bringing my lunch? That sounds like a boring alternative that doesn't thrill me too much. Help!

Norma Rae

Dear Norma,

I know what you mean. I find myself dreaming of cafeterias, and then the dream turns into a nightmare when I realize that very few of the rows and rows of foods offer things I should be eating. You stand in line at a cafeteria and get overwhelmed with the smell of everything at one time. Then you start seeing these foods that you never—I mean, never—make at home. Or you had something last week that was so good that you want to see if it's as good this week. You pick one of these and one of those and pretty soon you can hardly carry your tray. And then, on your way out of line, you pass the fourteen rows of desserts. Chocolate pudding pie with four inches of meringue. Strawberry shortcake that's as tall as I am. Berry pie topped with whipped cream in waves and ripples. You can't get past the desserts without taking one. Before you know it, you've spent $9.67 for lunch and have enough food for the entire factory staff right there on your tray.

The best way to get through a cafeteria line is with blinders on. Use mental blinders if you're not crazy about black satin. Do not see anything but the food you are ordering. Know what you're ordering before you get into the line, like soup and a salad. And never change your mind. Forget breads, desserts and goopy mayonnaisy salad dressings. You want a simple, nutritious, light lunch so you don't gain weight or take to sleeping on the job. You can do it, I know it.

Love,

Richard

Trap #4
Dear Richard:

Business lunches are part of my life. I have to go out with clients. I have to go out with my boss. Sometimes we have business entertaining in the evening right after a big business lunch. Then there's office lunches—someone's always leaving, or recovering, or having a birthday, or retiring, or getting transferred. There's conference lunches too. Almost all my work is done over a lunch table. Pretty soon I will be as big as that table. But I can't give up my job. Should I stop eating dinner?

Successful

Dear Successful:

I'm glad to know you're doing so well in your job. But if you keep up all the eating, you may not live long enough to enjoy your success. I know your problem and I know what you're going through. The day after you have a big business lunch you bring two carrot sticks and two celery sticks to the office in a brown paper bag as a kind of punishment lunch for what you ate the day before. Then, of course, you don't eat the punishment lunch (that would be a cruel and unjust punishment) but go out with some business associates and talk about deals. After you've eaten *that* lunch, you promise yourself you won't eat dinner so you can get back to your regular weight. But when you get home, you somehow manage to consume all of your dinner, including the butter, parsley, and lemon wedge on your plate.

There are several things you should be doing to survive your predicament. First of all don't look at a menu in the restaurant—order what you know is on your food plan. (If you go to a fancy enough restaurant, they will probably make something special for you.) Admit to everyone at the table that you think this kind of eating is crazy and get all your business partners to cut back on their eating. Then, instead of dessert and coffee and cigars and more business chat, pay the bill and go for a walk while you continue your discussion. Walk off some of that food and still get something done. You'd be surprised how far you can walk when you're having a good conversation. Miles will fly by without your noticing them. And at the end of the business meeting you will feel tremendously better.

Love,

Richard

WEEKEND LUNCHES

Five days a week you hack it out, nine to five, without so much as Jane Fonda, Lily Tomlin, or Dolly Parton to ease you through the week. You bring your lunch in a paper bag or a tin box, you stand in line at the company cafeteria to eat institutional food, you try various restaurants, or you live through a combination of all these meals. Then comes the weekend. Suddenly your routine is turned topsy-turvy. Your stomach goes into shock and your brain goes numb at the thought of what to have for lunch.

Well, rejoice, rejoice. Weekends are a celebration, not a problem. Weekends are the only time of the week that you can rebalance your food plan and take a look at your total weight and the problems you're having in controlling it.

• Weekends are the time to realize that you may have gone overboard during the week, so you can really exercise while staying on a strict food plan and get yourself back in shape for the weekend.

• Weekends are the time to splurge with something a little special for you and your family because you've been so careful during the week and you've got the extra time on the weekend to work off the extra calories.

So rise and shine, everyone. First thing Saturday morning I want you to have a family weigh-in. Use the chart in the back of the book to record your weight—and everyone else's—over a period of weeks. If your weight is down and you want something special, try one of our specialty breakfasts (see p. 42) on Sunday morning. If your weight is up, double your exercise program and slim down the size of your food portions. Go to bed hungry—but not without eating!—it won't kill you. And for goodness' sake, no weekend drinking! Beer, wine, and liquor are all fattening.

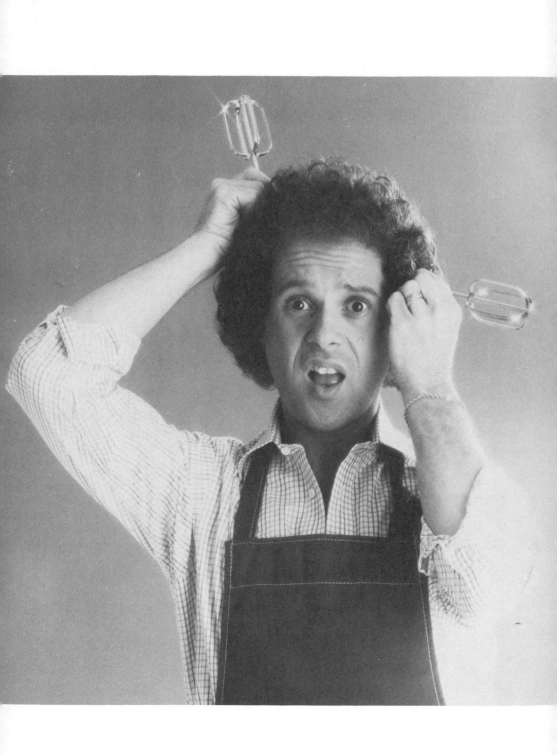

Teatime
and Other Daily
Crises

THE TEATIME TRIP

Okay, okay, I know all about it. It's four o'clock in the afternoon. This book is getting heavy. Your head is beginning to spin. Your back begins to ache and you're just plain wilted. You can no longer continue at your desk without a little respite. Or the kids are home, checking to see what Betty Crocker baked today, and you really think you should be with them even though their constant bickering gives you a headache at this time of the day.

What you need is a little nip. A zip of energy. A cup of coffee. A mug of tea. Some instant soup. A soft drink or two. A glass of wine. Anything to ease you through the end of the afternoon and make you feel alive again.

Your problem is not unique. Millions of Americans suffer just as you do. In fact, millions of people all over the world have the exact same feelings at the exact same time of the day. That's how teatime became popular, and later, cocktails.

You see, in most foreign countries, it is customary to take dinner at a rather late hour. They call it Continental Dining and no civilized person would consider putting soup to lip before nine P.M. These are the same people who ate a large meal at lunch and took a siesta at two before returning to work until seven. They made the long afternoon hours a little more comfortable by taking a break for tea at five P.M. Tea was not just a cup of warm brown water with one lump or two, but an elaborate arrangement that might consist of tea, coffee, or booze (or any combination thereof) and several types of cakes, biscuits, crackers, cheeses, and sweets. All these things were meant to fortify you until the late dining hour. It all became so involved that the English actually came up with High Tea and Low Tea. (Low Tea consists mostly of tea and maybe a morsel or two to chew on; High Tea allows for an array of goodies, including cake and sandwiches.)

Americans, who are always in a hurry (especially when it comes to meals), couldn't consider waiting until nine P.M. for dinner. They kept making the dinner hour earlier and earlier. From nine to eight; from eight to seven; from seven to six.

But they couldn't let go of their traditions either, and the idea of tea stayed with them. They just Americanized it by calling it Snack Time, and moved that back an hour, from five to four.

Snack Time became steeped in its own social customs—the four P.M. break coincides with the hour that children return from school. It's also the time that the television programming begins to turn from soap operas and movies to news programs and talk shows. The blood sugar runs thin, the energy konks out, and all of America is ready to shout for a fix of sugar or caffeine—or both.

And that's how junk food was invented. The British had their cucumber sandwiches—the Americans came up with candy bars. From candy bars it was all downhill: pizza, French fries, greasy burgers from a fast-food joint, milk shakes, tacos, root beer floats, crispy crunchies with salt on them, or popcorn coated with caramel and peanuts. No teen-ager ever seemed to walk into the house and shout, "Hey, Mom, I'm home. Have we got a few slices of lean turkey breast for me to snack on?"

After twenty years of junk food, American mothers decided to fight back and to supply themselves and their families with nutritious snack foods for the afternoon treat. Mothers grabbed their aprons, took to their kitchens, and began a series of elaborate preparations in which they researched recipes that yielded the latest fad foods. What are fad foods?

Fad foods are like fad anything else. You know how certain colors, certain clothes, and certain games become the rage, and you have a sudden need to be one of the first people on your block (but Heaven forbid, not the very first) to get into something new and kicky? Well, foods have the exact same kind of cycles. Some jet-setter someplace or another suddenly deems a new food to be "in," and the magazines and newspapers are suddenly printing lists telling you your foods are either "in" or "out." In order to stay "in," you spend an inordinate amount of time poring over fashion magazines, hanging out in fancy grocery stores, and using your midafternoon hours cooking (and sampling!) new concoctions that will prove to yourself, your family, and your friends that you are in with the "in" crowd.

One year it was jicama. Jicama is a Mexican root that is much like a potato but is great in salads and dips. It's only available in California and some southern locations. When jicama became the rage, New Yorkers were calling total strangers in Los Angeles and asking them to send them CARE packages by Express Mail. Then came spaghetti squash, and zillions of gullible people were suddenly—overnight—haunting their produce departments, their greengrocers, and their neighborhood Italian delicatessens, looking for spaghetti squash. (They were embarrassed to even ask if it was a vegetable or a pasta—it was so "in," they didn't want to appear "out" by not knowing.) Next came tofu. When I first bought tofu, I did the windows and the floors in my bathroom with it—I thought it was a sponge. Honest. I didn't know it was the rage. I'm so out of it.

The biggest problem with fad foods isn't that you have to spend a lot of time trying to keep up with the Joneses, but that cooks end up testing their fad food recipes late in the afternoon—before dinner and after the kids are home from school—and then they eat everything, thus gaining three additional pounds a week.

To see if you have a proclivity for such fripperies, I've devised a very simple little test. There's only one question in this quiz, so don't groan. It won't take too much out of you. But you have to be totally honest. Mark only your first response to this one question:

1. Kiwi is:

a. A type of shoe polish.

b. A bird from Down Under.

c. A fuzzy little fruit with green insides and little shiny black seeds.

See there, that wasn't too painful, was it?

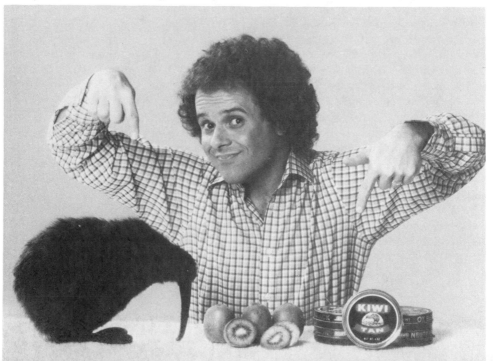

Scoring the test is even simpler, because all three of the answers are correct. If you chose answer (a) you're probably a sensible person with a good eye for the details of running a household or business. If you chose (b) you've a wild and exotic mind and read books about buried treasures and pirates and princesses. If you chose (c), well, it's out in the open: You're a snob, all right. You're into the latest fads and proud of it. You'll probably be serving your family the new Golden American Caviar within the next six months. (It's the latest rage, you know, at all the big Hollywood parties.)

Another hot new fad is fructose. I think someone has even come out with a fructose diet and a fructose cookbook. Fructose is a natural fruit sugar—it's about 70% sweeter than sucrose (table sugar), so a little goes a long way. This sounds reasonable enough, as if a magic cure-all for sweet-toothoholics had been found, and relief could be just a swallow away. There's just one catch. While fructose does have fewer calories than sucrose, once it's digested in the old body beautiful, the results are still the same. Every awful thing that sugar does to your digestion and your brain, fructose can do too. So you may not have gained a calorie or two, but you haven't gained anything else either.

So much for that fad.

C'mon now, do I see a tear in your eye? Are you telling me that if I take away coffee, tea, sugar, afternoon tea breaks, and junk-food snacks your life isn't worth living? Well, blow your nose—I don't want you dripping anything gooey on my book—because I've got a snack for you that's perfect for midafternoon, and I have this sneaky little feeling it's about to become the latest fad—hopefully a permanent fad—in this entire country.

It's called exercise.

What? Did I see you scrunch your nose up and roll your eyes? Did you dare to whisper under your breath that you're sick and tired of the idea of any more exercise? Well, spank your bottom.

I want you to take a look at this hard cold statistic and then tell me how you feel about exercise.

Of all the people who lose weight on whatever weight loss program they have succeeded with, 94% gain back that weight (and sometimes additional weight as well) within one year. One year. The 6% who keep the weight off keep it off not only for one year but forever because they have combined their food plan with exercise.

Exercise is the key to your salvation. And don't you forget it.

So far we've gone through the day together, and it's been pretty nice. You've gotten to eat some well-balanced meals; we took away your coffee break, but we gave you a social stimulant in its place; we haven't been mean or strict or nasty or rude.

So here it is.

Four o'clock in the afternoon is the perfect time for some strenuous exercise. And I mean strenuous. Go out and take an exercise class if you can. Sweat. Do some aerobics. Get your body working to its fullest potential. Then stretch that potential to newer heights.

If you work at home, I want you to take off your clothes (not right now, you can finish the chapter first) and put on a leotard or a bathing suit or a sweat suit and get to it. Turn on some jazzy music. Invite the neighbors in. Recruit the kids. Set the metronome. Shake it out, baby. Forty-five minutes of serious exercise will leave you more refreshed and revived than any sugar-coated pastry or cola or coffee-tea combination you could ever concoct. And after your workout, take a brisk shower, fluff up your hair, and take a good hard look at your naked body in the mirror. Assess your weaknesses and strengths. Be proud of your successes. Become more determined to conquer your problem areas. Then march into the kitchen and fix your family a Live-It dinner.

If you work in an office, this program just won't work for you. I'm not totally out of it! I know that the boss would frown if you stepped into a telephone booth, yanked off your three-piece suit, and revealed a navy and gray striped sweat suit. Management doesn't usually appreciate it if you walk off the job in the middle of a meeting because it's time to jog around the block.

But I'm not reversing my position. You need an exercise break. And you need a strenuous one. Depending on the formality of your office, try any of these suggestions:

If you work in the stuffiest of offices, where propriety is considered next to cleanliness in its closeness to God, hit the stairwells. When no other form of exercise is available to you, always remember the stairwells. I expect you to do two miles (get a pedometer) on the stairs in a walk-trot-and-jog pattern as you build up strength. You'll still have to do many other exercises at home in the morning or at night and on weekends, but this is a very healthful afternoon break for you. And you won't have to change your clothes. If you happen to be one of those people who sweats a lot, keep a clean shirt or blouse in your office.

If at all possible, convince your boss (or your employees) that production will increase after a healthful exercise break. Just as you organized your neighborhood, organize your office. I've already heard from people all over this country who are able to do this—factory workers, clerks, whole corporations, everyone. You don't have to break down into groups according to your pecking order in the company—we're all created equally, remember? So everybody get together and get out there for some serious strutting.

If it is impossible to do anything else, take a fifteen-minute break for isometrics. Just don't do too many of these exercises in a meeting with people you don't know too well. They might think you're real weird.

• Put your hands up (eye level) as if you're being arrested. Face the palms of your hand outward and pretend that two large walls of chocolate are coming at you and you are pushing them away.

• Inhale through the nose and slowly exhale as you push. Come on, push harder, or your head will get squished to death by the chocolate bars.

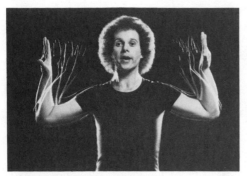

• After all the air has left your inside, return your hands closer to your ears. Inhale again, and this time push a lot harder as you exhale. Please keep your neck up and your stomach in.

• Repeat this exercise *ten* times.

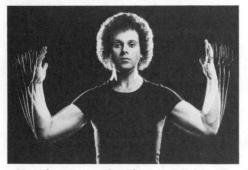

• Now keep your hands up and this time face the palms inward. It's as if some loud music is playing and you are trying to cover your ears, but something is holding you back (that something is the strength in your arms and chest).

• Inhale and start pushing in, but resist . . . resist more as you exhale. Donna Summer is screaming in your ears, but you just can't get to them.

• Repeat this exercise *ten* times.

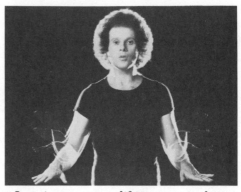

• Imagine you are lifting a very heavy box (no, not a fifty-pound box of candy).

• Inhale and push up with your hands as you exhale. You will feel a shaking sensation, but keep pushing upward until you're all out of air.

• Lift *ten* times.

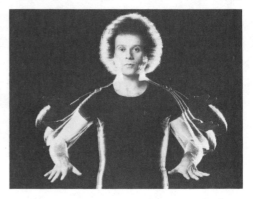

• Now you are pressing down on the box, so your palms are face down, of course.

• Inhale (is your stomach in)?

• S-L-O-W-L-Y exhale as you push downward.

• Repeat this exercise *ten* times.

During these isometrics remember at all times to keep a straight back and your chin up, relax the muscles in your face, and spread the fingers as wide as possible.

We've talked about constant movement in the body—well, the face needs constant correct movement also.

Will all the lines in your face and neck disappear? No. Can some of the loose skin firm up a bit and give your face more tone? Yes. Can you look years younger without surgery? Absolutely.

Let's Face It

Do you have to face it? No, not really. But if you have worked hard firming up the muscles in your body, don't you think the muscles in your face also need a workout?

Quick, get a mirror—and don't tell me you don't have one.

Look at your face and your neck. Well, what do you think? What's going through your mind as you stare at a big part of you? That you've neglected these areas?

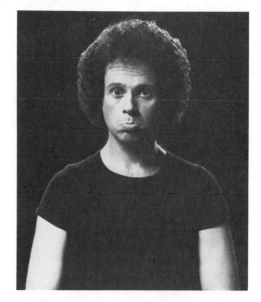

1. "It looks like a road map; where did all those lines come from?"
2. "I really don't know what happened. I look so puffy and distorted."
3. "I have to admit I look a lot better in pictures. Guess it's because all that light flashes in my face."

If you think gravity pulls down on your body, multiply that pulling force by ten and that's what's happening to that baby face and neck of yours.

Sagging skin and lines are indications that certain muscles are not being used.

Pout-ers

• Now hold your head up high and pout.

• Don't tell me you don't know how to pout—you didn't gain that weight by saying no. Like me, you usually pouted until you got what you wanted.

• You are now going to tone up your chin and mouth area. Inhale through the nose as you pout, then drop your chin all the way down and exhale through the mouth.

• Repeat the pout *ten* times.

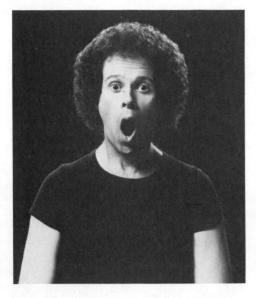

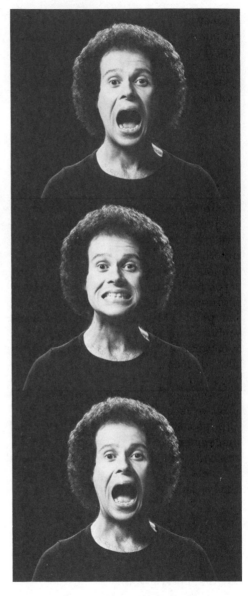

Chew-Man-Chew

• Head up again. This time open your mouth and start chewing (straighten that back and hold that stomach in. No one's at ease yet).

• Come on, chew wider, exaggerate a bit. You also didn't get that shape by taking small bites.

• Keep that head up and chew. This is the only time you have ever chewed without gaining weight. Air is very dietetic, you know.

• *Twenty-five* nice, big chews, please.

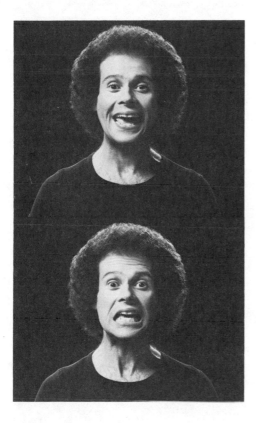

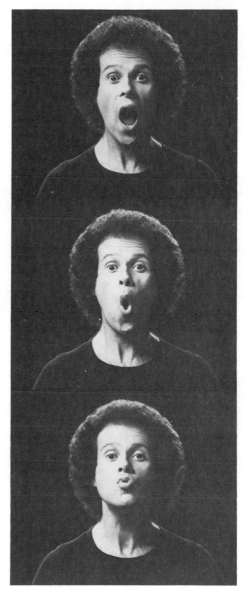

Vowel Stretchers

Remember A-E-I-O-U? They work all the muscles around your neck and mouth (and we know how important those areas are for eating).

• Look straight into the mirror, rest your eyebrows and forehead. Just concentrate on what's going on below the nose.

• Say the letter "A." It's a big smile, with your teeth a little forward.

• Hold your stomach in and get the sound of "A" out loud and clear.

• Inhale deep through the nose and exhale the vowel you are saying along with all the air.

• With "E" the corners of the mouth are pulling downward a bit, so most of your bottom teeth are showing.

• As you pronounce "I" elongate your face and drop your jaw.

• Pull all the way from your ears as you say "O." Start out with a big wide "O" and finish with a small one. Your jaw is still lowered doing the next vowel.

• "U" looks a little like a goldfish kissing the bowl. Your upper and lower lips protrude with your jaw and lower teeth pushed forward.

• So—you inhale through the nose and pronounce the vowels one by one while you exhale a little air out between them.

• Ready. Inhale and "A" (exhale) "E" (exhale) "I" (exhale) "O" (exhale) "U" (exhale). Good!

• Repeat *five* times and pay close attention to what's happening in the neck area. You are toning those muscles!

Under-Eye Tones
• This next one is so easy, you'll love it! It tightens the skin under your eye where bags and lines find a home.

• Close your eyes and relax all muscles on your face.

• While they are closed, without moving your eyebrows or forehead lift the eyeballs inside the closed lids upward.

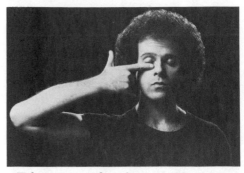

• Take your index finger and place it gently under the eye areas so you can feel the muscles working.

• Now keep those eyes closed and lift the inside eyeball again. Do you feel that pull? Well, that pull is toning up those under-eye areas.

• And you thought I was just pulling your eye.

• Be careful, now. Don't poke your finger in your eye, please.

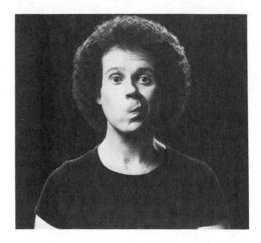

Wrinkle Wipes
• These aren't particularly attractive, but neither are chubby jowls and chubby

chins. Those small lines that keep getting deeper and deeper aren't so pretty, either.

• Your inhaling and exhaling will be done through the nose because the mouth is closed shut.

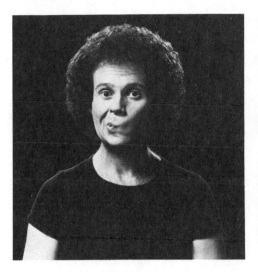

• Inhale and turn your lips all the way to the right side of your face. Hold it there and exhale. Inhale and come back to center, turn your lips all the way to the left side of your face, and exhale.

• *Five* wipes on each side.

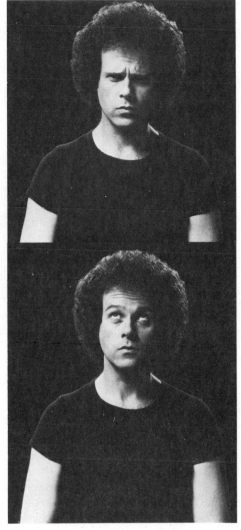

Frown and Stretch

• Pull your eyebrows down and close together. Hold for a count of three (one-two-three).

• Lift your eyebrows high and open your eyes as wide as you can.

• One of the reasons you get lines on your forehead is that you lift your brow and wrinkle your forehead more than the opposite pull, so the balance of your muscles is off.

• Set these straight and do *twenty-five* brow stretches.

Facial massages, chin straps, and clay—cement masks may bring the blood to your face and give it a glow, but only you can tone your face. Gravity does pull downward, and there are many other elements that cause wrinkles, lines, and over-all aging to the face and neck.

The sun. Isn't a tan pretty? Your skin is so brown and beautiful and dry! And when the tan fades away, what do you have? Right! Little teeny, fine lines—but they could be the start of something big. Because tiny lines become wrinkles in time. Sun blocks and suntan lotion, oils and creams help a bit, but anyone who adores the sun will get lines quicker than the ones who just don't make a big habit of lying out in those harmful rays for hours.

Wind, snow, and other weather elements. Also dry the skin and break down its elasticity. Since the skin on your face is a bit thin, you should protect it when you are out in bad weather.

Not wearing your glasses. And constantly squinting your eyes wrinkles your brow. Pulling your mouth up and distorting your smile lines makes for permanent indentations. If you hate your glasses, get contacts. If you hate glasses and contacts, you are in deep trouble and deep wrinkles.

Smoking. The mechanics of inhaling smoke from a cigarette causes tiny lines around your mouth area. The habit of smoking itself discolors skin, breaks down tissue fiber in your face and body, and doesn't do much for the whites of your eyes, either.

Drinking. Breaks tiny veins in your skin called capillaries. So little red lines run all through your face. Attractive, isn't it? Drinking causes puffiness around your eye area, and all that drinking is just no good for the pores.

Lack of sleep. Shows in your face more than anywhere else. There's no glow to the skin, no life, just a lot of bags and an overall droopy look.

Worry. Also shows first in your face. But after exercising your body and your face, what's to worry about?

If someone suggests you have a business meeting over cocktails (at what is sometimes called the Happy Hour, although the only people who get happy from it are the tailors who have to let out your clothes and the retailers who have to sell you larger sizes), countersuggest that you have the meeting in a health club or spa—someplace where you can both ride exercycles or sauna while you talk business.

When you're meeting a secret lover for a quick rendezvous, don't huddle in a booth in a dark corner of a bar—go out into the streets and mingle with rush-hour traffic. Walk in the crowds, and no one will ever notice you—or suspect a thing.

What's most important to remember is that when it's four o'clock, and you're thinking that the day is almost over, you're wrong. The new day is just beginning. Four o'clock is the Salvation Hour. Everything you didn't do earlier in the day can be corrected now. It's not too late. If you overate at lunch—it's okay. We all make mistakes. Take time after four to do some heavy exercising. If you've hunched over a desk without a break the entire day or done errands nonstop—think of four o'clock as your personal Happy Hour. Stop whatever you're doing and do something for yourself. You owe it to yourself to be the best person you can be. And without a body and mind-stimulating break at four, you are not fulfilling your potential. Relax. Breathe deeply. And do something nice for yourself. Just make sure it doesn't include something bad for yourself.

- ⊘ No coffee.
- ⊘ No tea; herb tea only.
- ⊘ No soft drinks.
- ⊘ No candy bars.
- ⊘ No pastries.
- ⊘ No fruits.
- ⊘ No cigarettes.
- ⊘ No alchoholic beverages.
- ⊘ No foods filled with sugar or caffeine.

JUST EXERCISE

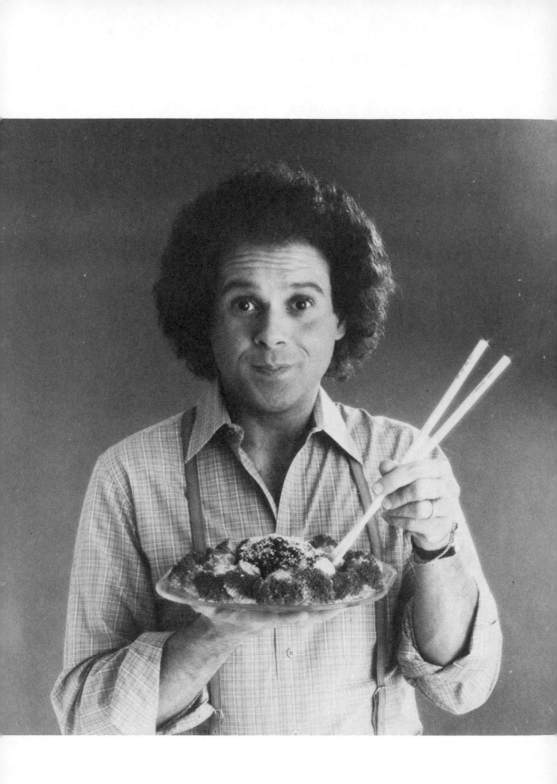

Live-It Dining

THE STORY OF D—
IT'S A VERY DIRTY STORY

You've heard about big D. Dallas. They call it a dirty town, filled with power and passion.

This is another story about big D. Dinner. You don't just have dinner in Dallas; you can have dinner anywhere, but it can be pretty dirty, filled with power, passion, and sometimes potatoes and gravy.

Why is dinner so dirty, you may ask. So ask already!

Because it was conceived in brown sauce, smothered in hollandaise, and destined to be served—course after course of it—at the end of the day when all folks had to do was lie back and bite in and gain weight.

Even the very basics of its name spell trouble. Some say the word *dinner* is derived from the Low Latin *di-coenare*, which in translation means "He who eats too heavy a dinner will die shortly of a coronary." The Romans fully understood this, since it was they who invented the word, and when they took over the running of civilization from the Greeks, they were quick to change the Greek habit of eating the heaviest meal of the day in the evening to eating such a meal between three and four in the afternoon.

Now, the Romans really did know how to pack it in. They ordered a meal in several courses: The first course was eggs and veggies (all served in vinegar, since there weren't too many preservatives and no Jolly Green Giants); then came a stew or roast; and finally pastries and jams, fruits and sweets. And that was just for the plain folk. At a Roman banquet—the kind when Ben-Hur comes to meet your folks—six or seven courses were served.

Throughout the Dark Ages the dinner hour shifted about. In France in the mid-1600s the heaviest meal of the day was served at midday, after Mass. But by the time of Louis XV, in say, 1770, the heaviest meal was back to late in the day. It obviously took Louis a long time to put on his wig, and he couldn't possibly appear for a noontime feast. And so it was that the French—thereafter considered the leaders in matters of cuisine—brought us back to the original late-evening dinner, which meant coronaries for all who wanted them. From then on the story just got dirtier and dirtier.

Dinner became more and more social. Men used dinner as a meeting time to discuss survival of the clans; they met to divide up the spoils of war and to celebrate the only two occasions worth celebrating: birth and death. (This was before Valentine's Day.) And in the process, the dinner meeting, the dinner party, and the banquet were invented.

DINNER SHOULD MEAN THINNER

There are people who tell you they hate to eat breakfast. There are people who tell you they never have time for lunch. But there is no one, no one at all, who will tell you he doesn't like and doesn't eat dinner. Dinner is America's favorite sport. Some people even give up watching TV to eat dinner. Others build entire social occasions around it. Family rituals and mating games have become intertwined with eating the day's last meal.

Not everyone takes his dinner in the same manner. There are a variety of different styles, and because eating dinner is such a social-familial occasion, these styles are passed on from generation to generation. Yet everyone falls into one of these categories:

1. *The I-Don't-Think-I'll-Have-Any-Dinner-Tonight Eater.* This is the most dangerous dinner eater of them all. He absolutely gorged himself at lunchtime—there's no question about it. And so there's a lot of guilt. The only way the conscience will stop beating like a drum is categorically to deny oneself the pleasures of another meal. The rationale is that if lunch was so big, it should even out by counting as two meals. The fact is that skipping dinner is bad for your body. But the facts don't seem to matter because the I-Don't-Think-I'll-Have-Any-Dinner-Tonight Eater always eats some dinner. He's just big on announcements. Then he smells and/or sees what's for dinner and decides, well maybe a bite of that and a

bite of this. Pretty soon this person is at the dinner table, eating a full meal and saying that tomorrow will be another day. Sure it will.

2. *The I'm-Eating-Light-Tonight-Honey Eater.* This is one of my favorites. The I'm-Eating-Light-Tonight-Honey Eater has every intention of staying on his food plan and actually thinks he is doing everything in his power to stay on it. He does eat a salad for dinner. But the salad is filled with olives and sardines and three heads of lettuce, and shrimp and avocado, and a creamy-rich sour cream dressing filled with four kinds of cheese that are absolutely mouth-watering and eye-tearing. Beside the fact that this salad alone is *not* a light meal and that it probably contains 2,000 calories (if you're into calorie counting), the I'm-Eating-Light-Tonight-Honey Eater is so self-righteous, thinking he's suffered by giving up a plate of beef stew over noodles, that after dinner he pouts for most of the evening and sneaks into the kitchen for snacks and bedtime nibbles.

3. *The I-Only-Eat-What's-on-My-Plate Eater.* This person has only one major fault. He's lying. He only eats what's on his plate at the dinner table and while others are looking. But all through the course of the meal he has been calculating exactly what has been left in the serving dishes and what is on each family member's plate. The I-Only-Eat-What's-On-My-Plate Eater is also a big one to volunteer to help clean up the kitchen. It gives so many more opportunities to eat leftovers. If the I'm-Only-Eating-What's-on-My-Plate Eater actually only eats what's on his plate—three cheers! Let's

just hope he keeps moderate portions on his plate and does his exercises regularly. He can Live-It forever.

4. *The It's - Familytime - Dinnertime - What's-New-with-You Eater.* This is a dangerous character. Dinner is his life. He saves all the news of the day so he can report it at the dinner table. He skimps on meals and snacks during the day so he can feel guilt-free about the huge meal he is about to eat. This is the meat-and-potatoes person. Now, I happen to know perfectly well that there's nothing wrong with being a meat-and-potatoes person— if you eat just a little bit of meat and potatoes. But the kind of meat and potatoes the It's-Familytime-Dinnertime-What's-New-With-You Eater eats is *heaps* of meat and potatoes. With gravy. And then he takes seconds. He also eats a roll or two with butter, some salad, two vegetables, and a dessert, followed by coffee laden with cream and sugar. Without a dinner like this, the It's-Familytime-Dinnertime-What's-New-With-You Eater would be forlorn—he is psychologically dependent on the event. His mind is more hungry than his body, and he craves the social nourishment more than the biological nourishment. He needs help fast.

5. *The It's-a-Free-Meal-so-Why-Not Eater.* This is a special breed of eater found usually among single women or executives with expense accounts. This is the person who is either taken to dinner on a date or is out to dinner for business reasons and therefore won't be paying for the meal with his hard-earned Yankee dollars. To this It's-a-Free-Meal-so-Why-Not eater, there are two thoughts: (1) I'll

order anything on the menu and eat as much of anything because it's free, so I might as well take advantage of this wonderful opportunity to stuff myself. (After all, tomorrow I'll go back to being Cinderella); and (2) I'll order a ton of food I know I can't eat and then I'll take the leftovers home so I can have another meal tomorrow. Two free meals—wow!

There does happen to be a right way to eat dinner, and it combines a few of the best parts of these characters with none of their bad points. (Natch—why pass on the bad stuff?)

6. *The I'm-on-the-Live-It Eater.* This person returns from work as tired and hungry as the rest of us (after all, he's human too) but with a special determination made of pride—an inner glow of self-confidence that comes from having gained control of his body. He may want a drink or a quick pick-me-up snack, but he doesn't give in to temptation. If his energy is lagging, he does some breathing and stretching exercises, often with the whole family, as a spirited kind of family adventure and joint activity. The togetherness and the brisk music uplift his spirits, and whatever feelings of exhaustion he had a half hour before give way to a second wind. Dinner is eaten at a beautifully set table, but served buffet-style with Mom serving each member of the family. Everyone gets a nice-size portion, but no seconds. After dinner no dessert is served. After the dishes are in the dishwasher, the family piles into the station wagon and drives to the neighborhood shopping mall. The kids race to the entry. The parents tag along, talking. Inside the mall everyone walks up one side and

down the other, window-shopping and sharing the day's activities. An hour later everyone is home again: The kids are preparing for bed, the adults may watch some television or read. No bedtime snacks are served. Just hugs and kisses. And the promise that tomorrow morning's confrontation with the scale will show no weight gain.

A WARNING ABOUT FAMILY–STYLE DINNERS

What are Family-Style Dinners?
Dangerous, that's what.

The term *family-style* refers to the use of large serving bowls that hold all the food for a group of people. Mashed potatoes for seventeen are lumped into one big bowl. All the string beans are in one copper chafing dish. And so on.

What's wrong with family-style?

Everyone eats too much food, that's what.

It may be a nice way to get acquainted with the members of your family by asking them to please pass the whatever-you-want. But unfortunately when family-style dinners are served, everyone eats way too much. (That's also *weigh* too much!)

Have you ever been to a truckers' truck stop? Well, I have. And it's not a pretty scene. Everyone sits down at a huge family dining table and you think "Gee, this is real nice and homey, and I get to make some new friends." You're having a great time, and then the food

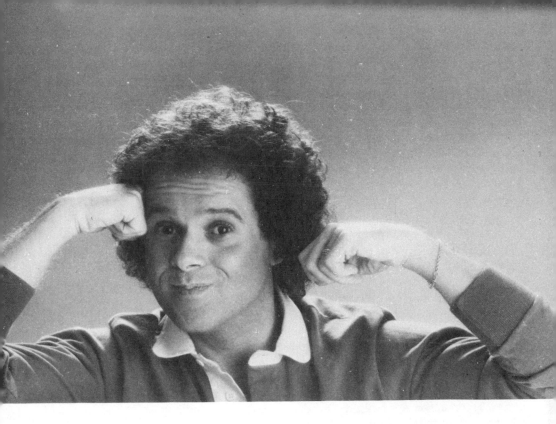

begins to parade out to your table. The iced tea is in a barrel as large as the ginger jars on my dining room table. The bowl of potatoes could serve the entire Chinese army. Cole slaw for two million arrives in a bowl the size of a wash basin. (It's more mayonnaise than cabbage, but it looks great.) Finally the fried chicken is served, along with biscuits and honey. The chicken comes out in baskets. Every-

thing is so deep-fried that you can't tell the chicken from the paper towels from the basket itself.

Then you get corn on the cob, and last but not least, your choice of three home-baked pies that are put right there in the center of the table so you can help your-self.

Are you beginning to see my point?

So heed this warning.

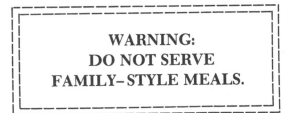

**WARNING:
DO NOT SERVE
FAMILY–STYLE MEALS.**

SETTING THE DINNER TABLE

I can see it now, as perfect in my memory as it was in person, fifteen years ago: our family dinner table. My mother was a big believer in making dinner a nice time of the evening. We had these cross-stitched tablecloths that my grandmother went blind making. With matching real cloth napkins that you were terrified to get dirty because then they would have to be laundered. We had this dinner china pattern, called Royal Chelsea, that was gold and white, and we had a double set—that way my mother didn't worry about breakage (actually my brother Lenny never ever broke anything, but well, I did), and you got more serving dishes. The number of serving dishes was very important to the scheme of our dinner table because we, like almost every other family in America, ate our dinners family-style.

These huge serving bowls matched the china and were continually passed around the Queen Anne dining table. The serving started with my father, who was very conservative and always took a small portion of food from the right-hand side of the serving bowl. Then the bowl was passed to Lenny. Lenny took his food from the bottom of the bowl—don't ask me how—but he did this neatly and quickly without ever messing up any of the food on top of it. Then finally, while I was drooling on my school uniform, I got the steaming platters and bowls. I always took the middle portion on the top because it had the most butter, the most cheese sauce, and the best of everything

else on it, and I wasn't stupid. (Or skinny, for that matter.) Mom took her helping from the side, always careful not to finish off the bowl, so there would be plenty of leftovers for seconds and lunch the next day.

After each bowl was passed, and your plate looked like the cover of some cookbook, we said a prayer thanking God for our day (and I always thanked Him for the extra serving platters too) and began dinner. All the serving dishes surrounded our plates so the table was one huge maze of dinner plates, silverware, glasses, napkins and food, food, food. Everywhere you looked, there was more and more food, and Peppy, my parakeet (he wasn't allowed on the bowls, though).

The dish set came with all kinds of extras—little jam pots and creamers and gravy pots—that you could buy a la carte—which my mother had bought two of. So all these extra accoutrements, which she claimed were the refinements of a proper dinner service, were also fit into the scheme of things on the table—laden with honey, hollandaise, condiments, cream sauces and everything else that might add to the tastiness of the meal. There was so much variety that it was imperative that you have at least two helpings of anything so you could decide if you liked it better with the cheese sauce or the sesame-tarragon mayonnaise whip.

After dinner my brother excused himself to do his homework (he was perfect!) and I helped Mom clear the table. I actually liked this job because it gave me a good opportunity to work over the leftovers that somehow disappeared on their way from the dining room to the kitchen. I was a human garbage disposal, but I called it helpfulness and wondered why I couldn't get a Boy Scout badge in leftover consumption. It took a long time to clear our dinner table because there were so many dishes, but this wasn't a task I minded, because it kept me that much closer to my good friend—food—and that much farther from my homework. And I was learning the basics of science and engineering. You see, early on I discovered that we had way too many dishes to fit on the kitchen counter if they were laid out side by side. So I began eating more and more leftovers off plates and serving bowls so that the dishes could be neatly stacked on top of each other without ever having to worry about improper balance. Who says you can't get an education in the kitchen? I probably should have become a civil engineer.

This went on until my eating became uncivilized. If your eating habits and dinner-table-setting habits are like mine were, you probably weigh as much as I once did. So let's relearn setting and serving. From the beginning.

RICHARD'S LAWS OF SERVICE

1. Set the table as nicely as you can. Placemats, tablecloths, matching dishes count. The meal is a special social occasion and should be treated as such.

2. Have a nonedible centerpiece: candles, flowers, a soup tureen filled with lemons. This will take up space on the table and still give the table a festive look.

The more room taken up by pretty things, the less room for serving bowls.

3. Have a pitcher of water on the table. Water is good for you. If you are tempted to ask for seconds, have half a glass of water instead.

4. Serve food in the kitchen. Do not serve family-style. Let one person dole out servings. Each person gets a healthy portion, and that's it, folks. (See list of portions, p. 204, to know exactly how much food we're talking about here.)

5. Never bring containers of food to the table. Besides being unsightly, it's too easy to eat everything in the container.

6. Clear all the dinner dishes before serving dessert. Matter of fact—everyone should bring his own dirty dishes back to the kitchen. It's no fun to eat a treat like dessert while looking at the battlefield remains of dinner. And the breather between courses gives you some time to digest and fill up a little bit.

Have the table-clearing chore rotate throughout your family. That way, if there is any cheating on the eating of leftovers, it won't all go on the body of one person in the family.

7. Do not eat off plates or out of pots and pans while you are putting away foods.

8. Put leftovers in well-marked containers. Small amounts of leftovers may be lumped together—if they're compatible—for a soup or stew at the end of the week.

9. Coffee does not need to cap off the perfect dinner. If you must, drink a decaffeinated beverage or some herb tea. If you haven't had milk during the day,

maybe a six- to eight-ounce glass of milk would be nice.

10. Do not eat dessert in front of the television set or "later on," which means before bed.

HOW TO FIGURE OUT YOUR DINNER MENU

I love it when people tell me that they go off their food plans because they couldn't figure out what to have for dinner. That's like opening up the closet to gobs of clothes and moaning that you haven't got a thing to wear. The problem in both cases is a matter of looking at the world with the right eyes. That old saying Grandma had about not seeing the forest for the trees often pertains. So let me take you by the hand, and guide you through the right way to plan a meal and stay on your volume food plan.

Begin all your meal preparations with one giant step for mankind. Clean out your refrigerator and your cupboards. Now, I know we've talked about this earlier in the book, but I'm repeating it now because it's so important. There's no reason for you to have anything in your house that you shouldn't be eating. This isn't Be Cruel to Animals Week. Give yourself a mental break: You won't have to wince every time you see a cake mix on the top shelf if there is no cake mix there. It's very simple. When alchoholics join AA, they just give up booze. I'm not about to ask you to give up food, but I am asking you to get rid of the wrong kinds of foods for you and your body and your

family. If you still don't know the right foods from the wrong foods, take a look back in Chapter 1 at Meet Your Live-It Foods. These are the foods you want to have in your home. You can forget the soft drinks, low-calorie fizz pops, frozen desserts, all those boxes of instant anything, foil-wrapped snacks, and the two dozen varieties of jams and jellies you like to have on hand to feel like a complete person.

Okay, now that we've got you cleaned and purified, you're ready to make the everyday decisions that affect you and your family. For the convenience of your grocery shopping, make out a rough menu for the week so you know what to buy in the store. Always shop with a list. You don't have to have complete menus chosen for all seven nights of the week if that's not your style—just know the basic food categories that are on your food plan and stock up. Your freezer should always have plenty of chicken in it. It should have no pork products in it. If you're planning red meat for your family, keep it down to once or twice a week if you can. Avoid packaged ground meats. Fresh fish is better than frozen.

Stock up on lots of fresh vegetables. You can buy for a whole week if you store the veggies properly. Frozen vegetables should be an emergency food and canned vegetables shouldn't even be discussed.

Now, then, when you go to make out your weekly shopping list, compare your daily foods to your proposed dinner menus. If you had red meat for lunch, you should not have red meat for dinner. Since there are probably several people in your family, and it's impossible for you to switch dinner around depending on what they all had for lunch, it's your duty to announce what the next day's dinner will be. Or you can post a note on the family bulletin board. (See the Poster for Tomorrow Night's Dinner in the back of the book.) And don't worry about that old wives' tale that you can't eat anything from the same food category twice in one week. If you had chicken on Monday, you may indeed want chicken again on Thursday—if the chicken is made an en-

tirely different way. Chicken happens to be a great food for the body and shouldn't be written off to once a week. Of course, if you have chicken for Monday dinner and leftover chicken for Tuesday lunch, then you certainly won't want it for Thursday dinner and Friday leftover lunch. But you don't have to go into the wrong foods in order to get some variety into your dinners.

Your weekly dinner menu plan should look something like this:

Weekly Dinner Plan

Sunday	boneless chicken breast
Monday	calf's liver
Tuesday	veal
Wednesday	fish
Thursday	Cornish hen
Friday	lamb steak
Saturday	Dinner out! Free choice.

Weekly Dinner Plan
Fill in your Live-It menus each week.
Remember: Variety counts!

Sunday	
Monday	
Tuesday	
Wednesday	
Thursday	
Friday	
Saturday	

I happen to eat liver every Monday night. But I don't eat veal every Tuesday or fish every Wednesday, on down through the chart. And I don't suggest that you yourself be so strict either. (C'mon, fess up, you wear the panties that say Friday on them on Tuesdays sometimes, don't you? Just for the fun of it?)

There are zillions of ways to prepare these foods so that you can enjoy the variety you need to stay on a sensible food plan. And every now and then you can splurge, especially if you're on maintenance, not weight-loss plans. But you do need to get rid of any extra splurging by exercising heavily almost immediately after overindulging. Don't call those pizza thighs cellulite when you know full well those little bumps are undigested pieces of pepperoni!

On the next page is a menu planner for next week. Try it. If you need some fresh ideas, you've come to the right place. This just happens to be a cookbook.

THE CHINA SINDROME

It's absolutely a sin. And I went to Catholic school, so I'm an expert on sin. So every night I say a prayer, and my prayer is that more people will discover Chinese-cooking techniques. Throw out your frying pans, sinners! Buy a wok. If you can't buy a wok, borrow a wok. If you can't borrow a wok (no no no, don't steal a wok, that's an even bigger sin), turn a skillet into a wok, but get rid of your old fashioned frying and buttering and learn to stir-fry and quick-cook.

Get a steamer. (The straw kind can catch on fire if you have a gas range, so be careful; I've seen some beautiful porcelain steamers.) Buy some chopsticks or ask your local Chinese restaurant if you can take yours home after dinner one night. And remember the essentials that have made the Chinese people so healthy: Go light on meats and heavy on veggies.

Some people complain that they enjoy their Chinese meals, and then two hours later they're hungry. For people who seem to have insatiable appetites, you can serve rice with the dinner—brown rice is preferable. Let people eat their meals and then have the rice if they're still hungry. You needn't serve the food on top of rice to try to bulk up the meal. One of the benefits of Chinese cuisine is that it's light. And its lightness also makes it a good choice for an evening meal when you don't want a seven-course banquet clogging your body before bedtime.

Not all Chinese food is on the Live-It plan. So don't go sending out to your local takeout place for several goldfish containers filled with food while feeling smug about your efforts to reduce. On the Live-It we have a few very scrutable rules:

Home-cooked Chinese is preferred to restaurant-cooked because you can control the ingredients better.

Use no monosodium glutamate in your home; in a restaurant ask the waiter to ask the cook to kill the MSG.

Use chopsticks whether you know how to manipulate them or not. Whatever food falls through is so much the better for your waistline.

Stir-fried dishes are great; crispy or twice-fried are not for you.

Soy sauce is high in salt, so just because you're not using salt don't think you've found the perfect flavor-enhancer.

Don't serve Chinese food family-style. (Don't serve anything family-style, remember?)

Apply the Live-It foods to your Chinese cooking. Pork is still a no-no. Chicken is still your best friend.

Go ahead and serve each person a fortune cookie after dinner. They're made of sugar but they're small, and they add such a touch of excitement to a meal that the extra calories are worthwhile.

Skip the MSG please.

FOR MOTHERS ONLY

Don't tell me, I've heard it before. Your five-year-old son (Jason? Joshua? Justin? Choose one, I know it's one of those) refuses to eat anything for dinner except macaroni and cheese—canned at that. He won't touch vegetables. He'd sooner die than try liver. And there's a good chance that if you don't give him the macaroni

he craves, he'll throw a temper tantrum and toss whatever else you're offering him right into your face.

If you get lucky, and offer it as a side dish to his beloved macaroni, just maybe you can get him to try something new. But you've got to be lucky; the moon has to be in the right position in the sky; the vibes have to be right; and a good bit of patient game-playing may be called for. The kind of games where you both make-believe that the fork is an airplane that is flying high; whirling left; twirling right, high, low; circling in and out; and finally somehow landing in your son's mouth. Hmmmm, ummmm. Isn't that yummy?

Or you may need to play another game. One for Jason. One for Mommy. In no time at all, Jason has eaten half of his dinner and Mommy has eaten the other half. Good for Mommy. She gets a gold star. And a big tushie.

So if you're the mom of a toddler, try some of these tips for size:

Don't force a child to eat or cajole him with games. He won't die of starvation if he doesn't eat this meal.

Scientific studies show that young kids eat what they need to eat, with or without your help.

Don't butt in. You can push your child to overeat. And then you'll have a *real* problem.

Children between the ages of one and two are far too interested in the world around them to concentrate on food. One good meal a day is all you can expect from them.

◖ Fat children become fat adults. Be thankful for picky eaters.

◖ If the child won't eat the food on his plate, write it off or give it to the dog. Don't *you* eat it.

THAT'S ENTERTAINMENT

This is a declaration of war. I don't care about the NATO treaties. I don't care about the Geneva Pact. I'm not asking for your sons—I'm asking for your sons, your daughters, yourselves, and everyone else you know. (Sorry, no pets.)

I am declaring a war on traditional entertaining. Not entertaining, mind you, just old-fashioned entertaining. The idea that you go to someone's house to stuff your face is disgusting. Here you are, doing perfectly well on your own Live-It, managing a sensible food program and then suddenly you go out to dinner, it's someone's birthday, you get invited to a cocktail party or a big family dinner, and you're wheedled and nagged to eat everything that's laid out on the table.

The legs of the table are bowed and the center sways under the weight of all this food, yet each guest is encouraged to put aside his objections and just this once, make like Miss Piggy. Not too many people know it, but you can have a great party and not serve food (or drinks) that are loaded down with the stuff that makes mountains out of molehills.

I'm not trying to tell you that on your birthday you should serve celery stalks with candles in them. I like a good time as much as the next person. What I am saying is that entertaining deserves to

change. Because you deserve better than what you're getting.

If you really like your friends and care about them, you should serve them foods that are good tasting and good for them. Any of the recipes in this book can be expanded for a company meal or party plan. If your friends have any respect for you—they'll do the same.

So the next time you go to a party, or give a party, try some of these tactics:

🦁 Work the party carefully. If it's not your party, play like you're the host or hostess. Talk to each person in the party. Do this with one drink in your hand. You can sip at the drink if you want to, but you may not refill your glass. And no fair sucking on the ice.

🦁 After you arrive at the party, say hello to the host and hostess, then excuse yourself and go into the powder room. Take off your clothes and look at your body in the mirror. What do you see? Kind of sloppy, huh? A few too many bulges? Yeah, I do know what you mean. Now put your clothes back on and go out there to the party. Smile, chat, visit with your friends—but remember what you saw in the mirror. Do you dare eat anything now?

🦁 If you find the buffet table so filled with fabulous foods that you know you cannot help yourself from stuffing your face, there is only one thing you can do. Take a good hard stare at the table, let your jaw drop no more than three inches, stretch your arms out full length and then pass out in a dead faint across the table.

This will render you unconscious, which will prevent you from eating, and will ruin the food for everyone else. They may not be amused at the time, but someday they'll thank you for it.

Before you lift any morsels to your mouth, take a good look around the room. Everyone is eating and drinking. Study each fat face, each pudgy hand, each jowl and double chin. Do you really want to look like them? You will if you eat that food.

Eat a little something before you go to a party so you won't be so hungry when you get there.

Never try to make a meal from the hors d'oeuvres just because they're free.

You don't have to finish everything on your plate. Taste, tell everyone how good it is, then leave half.

Don't go from a party right home to bed. Stop off someplace where you can walk, or do some exercises so you don't lie in bed like a dead tuna, feeding your fat cells.

Don't feel obligated to drink. If you do drink, try to cut back. Light wines are less fattening than Scotch and soda. There's an awful lot of sugar in drinks.

Don't carry your war too far or to such extremes that you make everyone miserable. One of the benefits of the Live-It is that you are allowed to splurge. You just have to remember to exercise it off later.

Chicken Broccoli Casserole

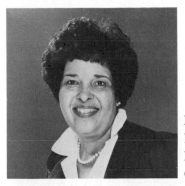

Name: Ruth Dyster
Highest: 230
Now: 166
Goal: 135

I'm Ruth Dyster, I'm an executive assistant in a film documentary series, and the Live-It is the only way I've ever been able to lose weight. I've tried everything—you name it, and I've tried it—shots, everything. But I'm real careful now. I eat a lot of chicken. I used to make Chicken Divan with brandy and mayonnaise. Now I've changed my old recipes around to comply with the Live-It. I'm real careful, since I sit at a desk all day. The only chance I get to exercise is morning and night, and I do that every day, but I also watch what I eat.

Ingredients

Serves Six

4 to 6 chicken breasts
sweet basil
1 bay leaf
2 tablespoons celery, chopped
2 tablespoons onion, chopped
1 pound broccoli, separated into florets

¼ cup water chestnuts, sliced
¼ cup nonfat dry powdered milk
1 tablespoon arrowroot
1 tablespoon sherry
pepper
brown rice

1. Wash, skin, and bone 4 to 6 chicken breasts. Cook in 1 quart of water seasoned with basil, bay leaf, celery, and onion. Cook breasts until tender, but not dry. Remove from liquid; reserve liquid.
2. Cut chicken into chunks. In a 2-quart casserole dish, layer chicken, broccoli, and water chestnuts. Layer until all ingredients have been used.
3. Make a gravy with 1¼ cups of strained chicken broth thickened with dry milk and arrowroot. Flavor with sherry. Pour over chicken-and-broccoli mixture. Cover with foil and bake in 350°F oven until hot. Serve over brown rice.

Catherine's Chicken Curry

Catherine can come cook for me any time.

Serves Four

12 large button mushrooms
1 teaspoon butter or margarine
1 clove garlic
1 large tablespoon chopped onions
2 whole split chicken breasts, skinned and boned

1 teaspoon curry powder
1 teaspoon dry mustard
1 teaspoon pepper
2 teaspoons tamari

1. In skillet, melt 1 teaspoon of margarine and sauté the chopped garlic and onions until golden brown. Place the mushrooms in the pan and let the garlic-onion butter absorb into the mushrooms. Cover and let steam to soften the mushrooms approximately 12 to 15 minutes.
2. Place chicken in a small baking dish and sprinkle with curry, dry mustard, and pepper and bake in a preheated 325°F oven for 30 minutes.
3. Remove chicken from oven. Place mushrooms under the chicken breasts. Sprinkle top of chicken with the two tablespoons of tamari to moisten the breasts.
4. Place back in the oven to bake at 375°F—yes, 50 degrees higher—for an additional 25 to 30 minutes.
5. Remove and serve 1 breast and 6 mushrooms a person, with its own delicious sauce of all spices.

From the kitchen of Catherine MacElveny

Designer Chicken

If nothing comes between you and your Calvins.

Serves Six

1 whole onion
3 chicken breasts, halved, skinned, and boned
1 cup chicken broth

2 tablespoons butter
salt and pepper to taste
¼ cup fresh lemon juice
1 tablespoon flour
2 egg yolks

1. Mince the onion and sauté in 2 tablespoons butter.
2. Brown chicken breasts lightly on both sides in the frying pan with the onions.
3. Add salt, pepper, and chicken broth. Simmer 30 minutes.
4. Add 2 egg yolks and 1 tablespoon flour to lemon juice. Pour over chicken and increase heat slightly for another 15 minutes. With luck the sauce and onions will boil down into delicious goobers to spoon over the chicken.

From the kitchen of Gregory Loeb

Mozzarella Chicken

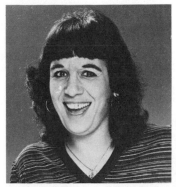

Name: Marilyn Lamas
Highest: 267
Now: 175
Goal: 130

I'm Marilyn, and I'm Richard Simmons' assistant, and he's saved me not once but twice. I've been heavy since I was 17. I broke up with this Marine I was engaged to and then I just pigged out. I never got thin again. I tried everything: pregnant-urine shots, hypnosis, pills. I've been to every diet doctor there is, and I've tried every gimmick to try. Then one night I was home watching television, and I saw Richard on *Real People*. I knew this was my last chance. I went to the Anatomy Asylum and when I walked in, Richard hugged me and I really got motivated right away. Richard said, "Stop smoking," and I did—cold turkey. I used to smoke 3 packs a day. I did what Richard told me, and I dropped weight. I've got 45 more pounds to go, and I know I can do it. Or he'll kill me. Anyway I was working in this office where all the people were heavy. I mean 300- to 400-pounders. When I started losing weight, they began to harass me on the job. It was awful. I began to get an ulcer, and my doctor told me to go on disability. Just then Richard rescued me and hired me to work for him. So he saved me twice.

Ingredients

Serves Four

4 chicken breast halves, skinned and boned
garlic powder to taste
1 tablespoon butter (or margarine)

2 cups tomatoes, peeled
½ teaspoon Italian seasoning
4 thin slices mozzarella cheese
1 tablespoon Parmesan cheese

1. Melt butter with garlic powder in nonstick pan, and brown chicken.
2. Purée tomatoes and add Italian seasoning and pepper.
3. Put chicken in baking dish. Pour tomato sauce over.
4. Put 1 slice of mozzarella cheese over each chicken breast and sprinkle Parmesan cheese on top. Bake in 350°F oven for 45 minutes.

Orange Chicken

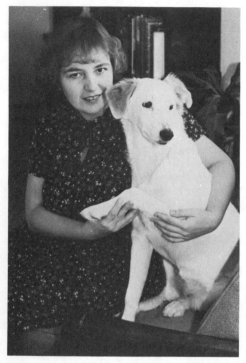

Name: Patricia Hyrman
Highest: 238½
Now: 178
Goal: 128

Hi. My name is Pat, and I was born in Marquette, Michigan, and I grew up heavy. I guess I always had a weight problem. I went on my first diet when I was 12 and oh, my word, I can't count high enough to tell you how many diets I've been on. At least 2 or 3 a year and you can multiply that out. I've never lost more than 30 pounds, but now I've already lost 60 pounds on the Live-It. What I like about the Live-It is that you don't need to eat diet foods. I like things that taste edible. I was never into nutrition or anything before, but I got involved with my little boy—he's 4—in trying to find the right foods for him so he wouldn't be heavy like I was. Then I got involved for myself too. I gained 30 pounds the first year we lived in Las Vegas (my husband's in the Air Force, so we've lived in a lot of places), and I'm just thrilled that I've lost so much weight. We cook a lot of chicken and have fish every now and then, and I exercise every day and go to a class here at the Nellis Air Force Base 3 times a week. My husband has been real encouraging—he used to bring me candy, but now he doesn't. Losing this weight is an adjustment for all of us, but we're coping. Now I just hope my mom will do the same thing.

Ingredients

1 2½- to 3-pound chicken, skinned, and cut in pieces
1¼ cup orange juice
1½ tablespoons tamari
1 tablespoon molasses
½ teaspoon dry mustard
½ teaspoon garlic powder

½ cup green pepper, diced
¼ teaspoon cinnamon
¼ teaspoon powdered ginger
2 tablespoons arrowroot
¼ cup water
1 orange, peeled and sectioned

1. Place chicken in 10-inch skillet. In mixing bowl, combine orange juice, tamari, molasses, mustard, garlic powder, green pepper, cinnamon and ginger. Pour over chicken.
2. Bring to boil. Reduce heat, cover. Simmer 45 to 50 minutes until chicken is tender. Remove chicken. Keep warm on serving platter.
3. Combine arrowroot and water. Add to remaining pan juices. Simmer 3 to 4 minutes until mixture thickens. Pour over chicken. Garnish with orange slices.

Saucy Plum Chicken

So tasty you won't believe it's chicken.

¼ cup chopped walnuts
1 egg, beaten
1 tablespoon arrowroot
1½ pounds chicken breasts, skinned, and boned
2 tablespoons sesame oil

1 cup fresh plums, peeled and puréed
1 1-inch piece of ginger, grated
3 tablespoons tamari
   green onions, sliced thinly
1 tablespoon sesame seeds

1. Pour boiling water over walnuts, let stand 5 minutes. Drain and pat dry.
2. Cut chicken into small bite-size pieces. In medium mixing bowl, combine egg and arrowroot. Add chicken pieces and mix well.
3. Heat oil in wok. Add chicken and cook on both sides until golden brown. Add walnuts and cook 1 more minute. Remove and keep warm.
4. Add plum purée, ginger, and tamari. Simmer for 3 to 5 minutes until sauce thickens.
5. Pour sauce over chicken, garnish with green onions, and sprinkle with sesame seeds. Serve over wok veggies.

Chicken Diosa

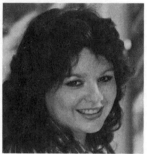

Name: Christine M. Price
Highest: 193
Now: 169
Goal: 110

I'm Christine Price, and I got so bored eating chicken that I had to come up with something new to help me stay on the Live-It. So this is Chicken Diosa. I made it up with a girl friend from work. I really love chicken, and this is something new. I can't eat red meat—it's too heavy. And I can't stand fish. So this is a recipe that's really helped me and my friends. I also exercise with Richard's TV show and I went to a spa. Whenever I get bored, I exercise by myself. Or I use the show as a warm-up, and then I do another hour's exercise. That and chicken can get you through!

Ingredients

Serves Four

2 chicken breasts, skinned, split apart
 and boned
⅓ cup white wine
 juice of 1 medium lemon

spices to taste: paprika, onion powder, garlic powder, parsley flakes, white pepper, poultry seasoning

1. Broil pepper-seasoned chicken 3 to 5 minutes on each side.
2. In casserole dish combine chicken, wine, lemon juice and seasoning to taste. Cover with foil.
3. Place on lower rack and bake in a 350°F oven for 40 to 50 minutes.

Chicken Sesame

Open Sesame and say Yum Yum.

Serves Four to Six

6 chicken breast halves, skinned, and boned
4 tablespoons soy oil
6 tablespoons sesame seeds
6 tablespoons tamari

3 large Italian squash, quartered and sliced
2 large onions, cut up
14 ounces (approximately) mushrooms, sliced
5 cups bean sprouts

1. Cut chicken into approximately 2-inch cubes or slices. Place 2 tablespoons of soy oil into wok or large frying pan and heat up. Place chicken and 4 tablespoons sesame seeds into hot wok or pan and cook about 4 minutes. Stir continually.
2. Add 4 tablespoons tamari. Cook approximately 4 more minutes or until chicken is done and sort of brown. Remove chicken and set aside.
3. Add 2 more tablespoons soy oil, add onions, and 2 more tablespoons sesame seeds and sauté. Add squash, mushrooms, 2 more tablespoons of tamari and sauté. Add bean sprouts and sauté.
4. Return chicken to wok or pan, mix all ingredients together, and serve immediately.

From the kitchen of Jan Welsh

Tarragon-Baked Cornish Game Hens

If eating is your game, you might be game for this one.

Serves Six

3 Cornish game hens, cut in half lengthwise
1 cup white button mushrooms
fresh garlic or garlic powder

brown rice
grapes
fresh parsley

Basting Sauce:

2 tablespoons lemon juice
1 tablespoon chopped fresh tarragon (or 1½ teaspoon dried)

½ cup white wine
¼ teaspoon freshly ground pepper

1. Mix basting sauce ingredients well.
2. Lightly rub each half of game hen on both sides with garlic powder. Place bone side down on a baking rack in a shallow pan. Place in preheated 375°F oven.
3. After hens have baked 20 minutes, drizzle sauce over them. Baste hens every 10 minutes with sauce from bottom of pan until the hens are cooked. Total baking time is about 1 hour to 1 hour 15 minutes, depending on size of the hens.
4. During last 20 minutes, put a cup of whole mushrooms in the sauce in bottom of baking pan.
5. Serve hens on a bed of cooked brown rice. Garnish with mushrooms, grapes, and sprigs of fresh parsley.

From the kitchen of Nita Bryant

Cheesy Halibut

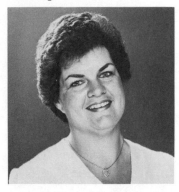

Name: Judy Melamud
Highest: 280
Now: 190
Goal: 140

I'm Judy, and I've lost almost a hundred pounds. I Live-It every day with Richard, and this is the easiest diet I've ever been on—and believe me, I've tried them all. I started gaining weight about 12 years ago when my daughter was born. But it took me until the spring of 1981 to get my weight under control. I exercise 2 times a day at least, and sometimes 3 times. I get great compliments from people who have seen my progress, and that's what keeps me going. I've been amazed at how fast the weight's come off. When my clothes start getting baggy, I get real happy. I eat a lot of fish, at *least* twice a week. At first I was cooking it with lemon, like Richard says, then I started goofing around in the kitchen and came up with something fancier.

Ingredients

Serves Five

1 tablespoon butter
1 medium onion, chopped
1 stalk celery, chopped
1 cup mushrooms, sliced
½ cup chopped parsley
½ green pepper, chopped
   dash of paprika

¼ teaspoon pepper
1 cup Cheddar cheese, shredded
3 tablespoons Parmesan cheese,
   grated
2 1-pound halibut steaks
   lemon wedges
2 tomatoes, sliced

1. Sauté onion, celery, parsley, green pepper, and paprika in butter until onion becomes translucent. Add mushrooms, sauté 2 to 3 more minutes.
2. Sprinkle each fish steak with pepper. Place fish steak in buttered baking dish; spread mushroom mixture over fish. Top with remaining fish steak. Sprinkle with Cheddar and Parmesan cheeses.

3. Bake in 400°F oven for 20 to 25 minutes, until fish flakes easily when tested with a fork. Place on serving platter. Garnish with lemon wedges and sliced tomatoes.

Shrimp-Stuffed Flounder

Make this one when your mother-in-law comes for dinner.

Serves Four

4 ounces baby shrimp, cooked	1 teaspoon chopped chives
1 egg, slightly beaten	2 teaspoons flour
½ cup skim milk	2 8-ounce flounder fillets
1 tablespoon butter	2 tablespoons dry sherry
	white pepper, paprika to taste

1. Mix shrimp, egg, and ¼ cup milk. Melt butter in skillet. Sauté chives 1 minute. Add flour and cook till bubbly. Add shrimp mixture and cook till thickened.
2. Split flounder, either by making a pocket or cutting them in half. Fill pocket with shrimp mixture and close with toothpicks.
3. Pour remaining milk and sherry over fish. Sprinkle with seasonings.
4. Bake in 300°F oven for 30 minutes or until fish flakes easily when tested with a fork.

South-of-the-Border Snapper

Pancho Villa's fave.

Serves Six

6 red snapper fillets	½ onion, chopped
3 tablespoons fresh lime juice	2 tablespoons olive oil
pepper	3 cups fresh tomatoes, peeled and
2 green peppers, sliced	chopped
2 cloves garlic, minced	8 olives, sliced thin

1. Preheat oven to 375°F. Sprinkle both sides of fillets with lime juice and pepper. Put in refrigerator for an hour or so.
2. In big skillet, sauté onions and garlic in oil until soft. Stir in tomatoes, olives, and green pepper. Cook until boiling, then turn down the heat and simmer for 10 minutes.
3. Drain any water from fillets and put them into shallow baking dish in one layer. Pour tomato mixture over fish and bake for 25 minutes.

From the kitchen of Idrea Lippman

Crispy Fish Bake

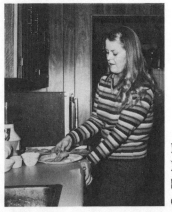

Name: Pamela Ross
Highest: 235
Now: 150
Goal: 130

I'm Pam, and I weighed 190 pounds when I left high school about 9 years ago. I started taking diet pills in high school, and for 2 months I was losing weight and doing great. Then I went off the pills and gained the weight back. I actually started to get heavy when I was 8. Before that, I was small and anemic. Then they took out my tonsils, and I gained 50 pounds in 6 months. After that I always said that they made my throat bigger so the food could get down easier. But now I'm on the Live-It. I exercise 2 times a day. I really don't like fish, except for real deep-fried or oil-packed tuna, so when I came up with this recipe, I knew I had a winner. If I like it, you know it's good. We eat very little red meat now. It's not good for you and it's so expensive, I'm glad to find some kind of fish I like.

Ingredients

Serves Four

2 pounds red snapper fillets (or any fish you prefer)
½ teaspoon salt

½ cup cornmeal
2 tablespoons buttermilk
lemon slices

1. Wash fish fillets and cut into serving-size pieces. Dip fish in buttermilk.
2. Add salt to the cornmeal and stir.
3. Roll fish in the cornmeal mixture to coat lightly. Place on an ungreased cookie sheet and bake in 400° F oven for 20 to 25 minutes, turning once at midpoint. Serve with lemon slices.

Salmon Puff
Puff the magic dragon has nothing on this dish.

Serves Six

6 ounces fresh salmon, steamed or
7¾ ounces canned salmon,
undrained
2 large eggs, lightly beaten
1 tablespoon chopped parsley
2 tablespoons onion, minced
2 tablespoons lemon juice
1 teaspoon prepared mustard
14 unsalted saltine crackers, crushed *or*
3½ pieces whole grain bread, dried
and ground into fine crumbs

1 cup low-fat milk
1 tablespoon butter, melted
dash salt
freshly ground pepper
dash Tabasco sauce
1 to 2 teaspoons dillweed
parsley for garnish
lemon slices

1. In medium bowl, break up salmon. Add all remaining ingredients. Mix well.
2. Turn into a 8- by 4- by 3-inch loaf pan or small pie plate.
3. Bake in 350°F oven 45 to 55 minutes or until puffed and center is set.
4. Cool 10 minutes and loosen from sides with a sharp knife. Turn out and place on serving dish. Garnish with parsley and lemon slices.

Shrimp and Scallops
Even fish haters should try this one.

Serves Four

1½ cups uncooked long-grain brown
rice
2 tablespoons oil
1 medium onion, chopped
3 fresh tomatoes, chopped
½ bell pepper, chopped
3 cups chicken stock

1 shot Tabasco sauce (or more, if you
like it hot)
1 cup shrimp
1 cup scallops
parsley
lemon slices

1. Put oil in pan and lightly brown the rice. Add tomatoes, onions, bell pepper and sauté 3 to 5 minutes.
2. Add stock and Tabasco. Cover and cook 45 minutes over low heat.
3. Add shrimp and scallops and cook 15 minutes or until rice is done.
4. Garnish with parsley and lemon slices.

Green Bean Bake
From the valley of the ho ho ho.

*Serves Four**

1 pound fresh green beans, French
   cut
2 tablespoons slivered almonds

⅔ cup kidney beans
½ medium onion, sliced thin in circles

1. In 1½-quart casserole, place half the green beans. Top with almonds, onion, and kidney beans.
2. Top with remaining green beans. Cover and bake in 400°F oven for 45 minutes or until beans are *al dente*.

*Serving size—½ cup.

Spinach Roll-Ups
Popeye's favorite dinner.

Serves Five

10 whole wheat lasagna noodles
 3 bunches spinach, stems removed,
   chopped
 3 tablespoons Parmesan cheese,
   grated

1 cup low-fat cottage cheese
½ teaspoon nutmeg
1 cup onions, sliced
2 cups grated Muenster or Jack
   cheese

Sauce:
4 cups tomato sauce
2 cloves garlic, minced or crushed
½ teaspoon basil
1 teaspoon oregano   *or* 2 teaspoons Italian seasoning
½ teaspoon marjoram

1. Cook and drain noodles according to package directions.
2. Steam the spinach until it is limp. Add the cheese, cottage cheese and nutmeg.
3. Spread noodles with spinach filling, roll up, and stand on end in oiled 9- by 13-inch baking pan.
4. Sprinkle cheese and onions on top of noodles. Combine sauce ingredients and pour sauce over noodles.
5. Bake in 350°F oven for 45 minutes or until tomato sauce is bubbling.

Rolled Sole Amandine

Roll over Neptune, this fish is fresh.

Serves Four–Six

2 cups mushrooms, thinly sliced
3 tablespoons butter
2 pounds fillet of sole
1 cup Mock Sour Cream (See p. 161)
²⁄₃ cup finely chopped almond slices

⅓ cup dry white wine
juice of 1 lemon
lemon wedges
freshly ground pepper
parsley

1. Sauté mushrooms in 1 tablespoon butter. Set aside.
2. Cut fish into approximately 3½- by 3-inch pieces. Place a small amount of mushrooms on each piece. Roll fish around mushrooms. Secure with a toothpick.
3. Dip each piece in Mock Sour Cream (See page 161). Then roll in almonds.
4. Melt 1 tablespoon butter in saucepan. Sauté fillets until golden. Add remaining butter, turn, and sauté slowly until fish flakes easily when tested with a fork. Remove and keep warm.
5. Add wine and lemon juice to pan drippings. Heat through. Pour over fish.
6. Garnish with lemon wedges and parsley.

Creamy Cauliflower

More than cauliflower makes this dish great.

Serves Six to Eight

1 tablespoon vegetable oil
1 large onion, chopped
¼ bell pepper, chopped
¼ cup zucchini, chopped
½ clove garlic, mashed

2 cups cauliflower florets
½ teaspoon dill weed
½ teaspoon marjoram
dash of nutmeg

1. In medium skillet, heat oil. Add onion, bell pepper, zucchini, and garlic. Sauté over medium heat until tender.
2. Steam cauliflower florets until tender. Combine cauliflower, sautéed vegetables, and seasonings in blender or food processor. Mix until well blended.

Eggplant Casserole

Eggsciting dish for vegetarians.

Serves Four to Six

1 large eggplant
8 whole grain crackers, crumbled
1 or 2 eggs

½ cup low-fat milk
1 cup grated Cheddar cheese
pepper

1. Peel and dice eggplant. Boil until soft and then mash. Add egg, 6 crackers, ½ cup milk, and pepper to taste.
2. Place half the mixture in a casserole dish. Add half the cheese. Now add the remaining half of eggplant mixture and top with the remaining cheese, pepper, and 2 crumbled crackers.
3. Bake in 350°F oven for 30 minutes.

From the kitchen of Skipper Johnson

Eggless Egg Rolls

A gourmet treat for everyone in your family.

Serves 4

4 6-inch square egg roll wrappers, cut
in half diagonally

Sauce:

3 tablespoons sesame oil
2 tablespoons tamari
1 tablespoon fresh ginger root, peeled
and grated

1 teaspoon sherry
1 clove garlic, mashed or minced
2 teaspoons toasted sesame seeds
½ teaspoon cornstarch

Combine in small bowl, set aside.

Filling:

2 tablespoons sesame oil
1½ cups shredded cooked chicken
1½ cups bean sprouts
1 cup bamboo shoots

½ cup water chestnuts, sliced
¾ cup green onions, chopped
hot mustard (optional)

1. Heat 2 tablespoons oil in wok or large skillet. Stir-fry chicken for 1 to 2 minutes. Add remaining vegetables for filling. Stir-fry another 2 to 3 minutes.
2. Stir sauce ingredients and pour over filling. Mix well. Remove from heat.
3. Place about one eighth of mixture in center of wrapper. Fold opposite corners in, then roll up wrappers beginning at the long edge. Seal tip with a drop or two of water.
4. Using additional 1 tablespoon oil, lightly brush both sides of rolls. Bake in 350°F oven until golden brown, turning once. May serve with hot mustard.

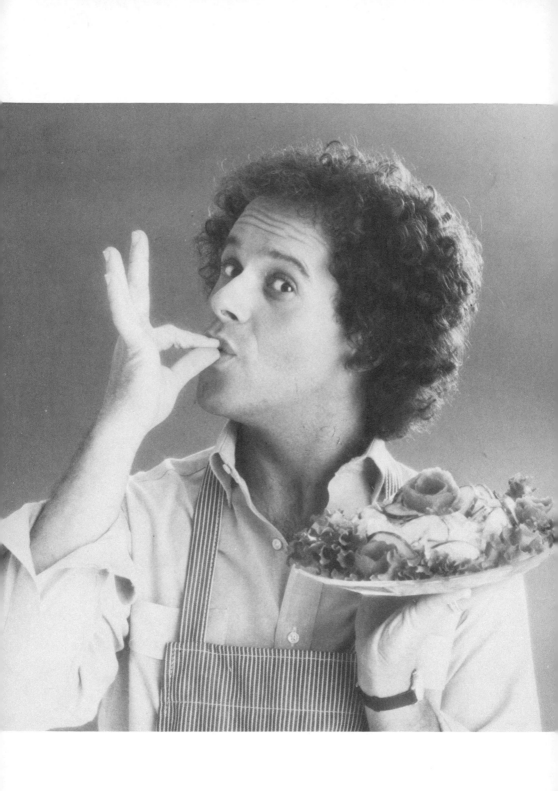

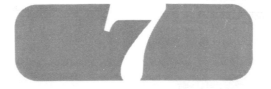

Not Just Another Head of Lettuce—Not Just Another Bowl of Soup

NOT JUST ANOTHER HEAD OF LETTUCE — SALAD DAYS AND SALAD NIGHTS

Have you ever heard the expression "It was in my salad days"? It's kind of a cliché that's supposed to mean that once you were young and poor and forced to eat salad, and it implies that once you got it together, you ate meat and potatoes, caviar and sour cream.

So right now I want all of you to do history a big favor. Would you please stop using that expression? I mean, if you're planning on losing weight or maintaining a weight loss, your salad days (and salad nights) are here—and you should be proud of it! You shouldn't aspire to meat and potatoes in the first place. Okay, for a treat every now and then; in moderation once in a while. Who am I to say no? But day in and day out, night in and night out, a salad is going to be your best friend.

And this is not some high-handed new remark. Long, long, long ago (I mean *really* long ago) salads were the only thing eaten at all. Because if you remember your history, you'll remember that many dinosaurs were salad lovers! So salads have a long and healthful tradition behind them. They were obviously a better idea than dinosaurs, because salads lasted, and dinosaurs didn't.

Salads have indeed lasted throughout the ages of man. They've changed with the times (haven't we all?) but they always reflected the attitudes of the particular time and the availability of foodstuffs.

Let's just take a look at our heritage of salads so we can see what a legacy has been left to us by people smart enough to know that man cannot live by bread alone.

The Tossed Salad: Not such a good idea. Was thrown out of the cave in 12,567 B.C. and thereafter called Tossed Salad.

The Caesar Salad: Invented in Roman times and dedicated to the ruler. Consists of lettuce, grated cheese, anchovies and a few croutons. Was once served on crushed ice gathered from hailstorms (Hail, Caesar!) and was a favorite meal of gladiators because it was filling but light enough to please.

The Ambrosia Salad: A fruit salad mixed with a creamy dressing and marshmallows that originated in rural Greece at the Temple of Ambrosia where the handmaidens spent their hours playing the lyre and making salad. Often dedicated to the god of sticky white treats.

The Greek Salad: Not to be confused with the Ambrosia Salad but also of Greek origin. This salad was invented centuries later by outer-island fishermen who had a yen for goat cheese and sour olives.

The Niçoise Salad: Invented by a French sailor's wife (named Nicole) who got sick and tired of tuna salad the way everyone else in her village served it and decided to come up with a better solution to the age-old problem of tuna, tuna,

tuna, I just can't get you offa my plate. Or palate.

The Fruit Salad: Originated by Eve (the one, the only) but not popularized until California was discovered.

The Potato Salad: A favorite of peasants everywhere, this salad was cultivated in the Dark Ages when few foodstuffs were available and one considered himself lucky to get a boiled potato for a meal. When one was so sick of potatoes that he no longer considered himself lucky to get a potato for a meal, he got potato salad.

The Chef's Salad: Originated for the Chief of Police in Philadelphia in the late 1800s and transformed into *chef* instead of *chief* through the misinterpretation of the local accent. Usually includes slices of ham, turkey, chicken, roast beef, and several cheeses. On the whole I'd rather have a chef's salad.

The Waldorf Salad: Invented by a waiter at a fancy New York hotel who later went on to establish his own Park Avenue hotel, still famous today, though now owned by the Hilton chain. Walt Dorf, in his early days, inadvertently confused a dinner salad order with a side order of sliced apples, and a trend was begun.

The Spinach Salad: Comic-book promotional salad intended to get Popeye to eat fresh spinach rather than canned. Includes spinach leaves, sliced mushrooms, crumbled bits of bacon, and sometimes some hard-boiled egg.

The Salad Bar: Introduced in Chimoya, New Mexico, in 1960 in a restaurant located too close to a church to have a liquor license but in desperate need of attracting patrons to some kind of bar or another.

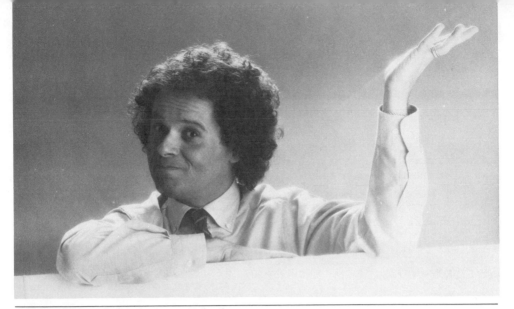

What You Can Put in a Salad

What to put in a salad:
(Choose one or all, in combination with lettuce.)

anchovies
apples
artichoke bottoms
asparagus
avocado
bean sprouts
beets
broccoli
brussels sprouts
cabbage, red or green
capers
cauliflower
celeriac
celery
cheese
chicken
chopped chives
chopped nuts
cooked vegetables
corn
cucumber
eggs

endive
fresh fruits of your choice
garbanzo beans
green beans
herbs
jicama
lean roast beef
mandarin orange slices
mushrooms
nasturtium flowers
olives
peas
pimientos
pumpkin seeds
radish
rice
sautéed livers
scallops
shellfish (go easy on shrimp)
spinach
sunflower seeds
sweetbreads (just a suggestion)
tomatoes
truffles
tuna
watercress

What not to put in a salad: (Choose none of the below.)

automobile parts
cookies—homemade or otherwise
Jell-O cubes
leftover gift wrap
marshmallows

old tennis shoes
pepperoni
pet food
pork products, such as ham, bacon, or sausage
salami
shredded paper
wood pulp

Best-Dressed List

I have a personal attachment to salad dressings. When my mother was pregnant with me, she was careful to eat a lot of fresh vegetables and eat a salad every day. Her salads were always smothered with Thousand Island dressing. I know this because when I was born, the doctors and nurses were shocked to see that I would not take to bottle or breast unless there were a few dollops of dressing added.

So from the beginning we were a very creamy family. Mother and her Thousand Island, Dad and his blue cheese; and me, I'd take creamy anything. Creamy Ranch was my favorite, but I wasn't real picky as long as the dressing spread rather than dripped. My brother Lenny wouldn't eat salad dressing at all until he was twelve, and then he ordered it on the side. (Oil and vinegar, of course.) But I always thought the salad dressing was the best part of the salad.

In a restaurant I used to say to the waitress, "And I'll have the dinner salad please; kill the lettuce, go heavy on the cukes, and flood it. Thank you." I had no interest in lettuce whatsoever but did

have a dedicated fondness for cucumbers. And salad dressing.

I discovered dietetic dressings in my teen years. Teen-agers, I'll have you know, don't really have skin problems. Unless they use dietetic dressings. The dressings always come in these cute little tinfoil or plastic packages—so the manufacturer can charge more while claiming you can only use this measured amount on this one salad—and while you're trying to open the package, it finally spurts out into your face. If you had that many chemicals and oil applied to your face regularly, you'd have pimples too!

All those diet foods came out in the 1960s, and as far as I'm concerned, they could have spent more time putting monkeys into orbit than letting the scientists of the world come up with these awful foods. It's just bad public relations. Crummy low-calorie dressings make people think that there are no good-tasting low-calorie dressings. And that's just not true. Which I'm about to prove to you.

But before we get into the good news about low-calorie dressings, let's just talk a bit about old-fashioned salad dressings. Most salad dressings are made of the kind of ingredients that go directly from your tongue to your heart, where they have a very big convention. When enough globules of olive oil, mayonnaise, and sour cream unite, you will keel over and have a heart attack. Just *TIMBER*, like the loggers shout. Watch out below, here comes another one!

Killer dressings, believe me, are a lot more prevalent than killer bees. Just walk into a restaurant—or take a quiet look around your own family dinner table—to see how people are stuffing their faces with gobs and gobs of grease. And usually they're very self-righteous about it. People who eat salad think they are helping out their bodies, think they are doing themselves and mankind a big favor. They actually think they are controlling their weight problems. The fact that the vegetables can't even breathe because of the 3,154 calories in the dressing is a mere technicality to them.

In order for the salad to do you any good, it must be topped with the right amount of the right kind of dressing!

Amount is important here. Let's face it, when the chafing dish has just tipped over and your tablecloth caught on fire and you can easily douse the blaze with the liquid from your salad bowl—you've got too much dressing on hand. So you have to watch the amount of dressing you use. But you also have to be aware of the ingredients that are in the dressing. And the ingredients in homemade dressings are better for you than the ones in store-bought.

Most people prefer store-bought dressings. They know they're missing a little on taste, but they think that the time saved is worth the compromise. It really takes about two minutes to make a home-made dressing (and that's two minutes toward a better and longer life) but most people would prefer spending two seconds sweeping clean the grocery store shelves.

The shelves are well dressed, I have to admit that. About five or six shelves, stretching for almost a third of the length of the grocery store, stock the varieties of dressings—the forty-seven varieties of oil are farther down, along with all the vinegars, the olives and for some reason, the popcorn.

The salad dressing rows are beautiful. There are bottles sculptured by glass-blowers in Greece. There are bottles created to look like Baccarat crystal—fine enough to place on the dinner table at the White House. There are wide-mouth bottles so you get more of the stuff out faster. There are jars rather than bottles, so you can get a serving spoon right into them. And they all have labels. Some have glorious colored pictures of the dressing being poured, so you can see how thick and creamy and drippy and yummy it is. Some show a picture of a salad, and instead of the lettuce looking soggy with all that dressing, the entire salad, dressing and all, sparkles and has flashes of light reflecting off of it as if the photographer were shooting diamonds in sunlight. The jars are the ones that go for the old-fashioned labels—using brown kraft paper and simple homey typefaces with a sketch or something of grandma to convince you that this dressing is the real McCoy.

Then there are the packaged salad dressings. These are my favorite because some of them come with little glass bottles and you think you're getting the bottle for free if you just buy the two packets of dressing. Then once you've got the bottles at home, you keep buying more and more of the packs. Over the last year or so I've noticed that there's a big red seal on the package that says NEW! IMPROVED! and I'm dying to write that company to see if the salad dressing has been improved or if the quality of the bottle has been improved.

These packaged dressings are very sneaky because even though they take just as long to make as dressings from scratch, you buy them in the store thinking you have (a) saved time and (b) made a homemade dressing. Now, that's what I call smart marketing. The real truth is, you fell for a pretty package, a Madison Avenue ad campaign, or some tricky strategy.

My favorite of all these kinds of dressings are the ones that say SECRET INGREDIENTS on the label in real fine print, as if this were an old family recipe and the company's livelihood would be diminished if you got their secrets. The truth is

they don't dare tell you their secrets because then you wouldn't buy the dressing: Who would choose to eat chemicals, preservatives, additives, and food coloring if he didn't have to?

Almost all salad dressings are the same, you know. You combine an oil with an acid and then add a few spices for taste. Commercial dressings also have stabilizers in them so they don't rot on the shelf. (It's so unattractive to find mold growing out of the bottle, don't you think?) While the preservatives do increase shelf life, there's a good chance that a substance called EDTA has been used, and this junk has been directly related in medical research to kidney damage. Real nice, huh? And you were eating a salad to get *healthy*.

So take some friendly advice from your old friend Richard. Forget about bottled, jarred, and prepackaged dressings. Make your own. And when you're shopping for the ingredients, if you must use oil, use peanut oil or safflower oil. Both are excellent all-purpose oils and have none of the chemicals you'll find in corn or other oil.

Fruit Salad Topping

It's the tops.

Serving Size: One-Half Cup or Four Servings

¾ cup plain low-fat yogurt
1 teaspoon honey
1 teaspoon grated orange peel
1 teaspoon grated lime peel

¼ cup orange juice
2 teaspoons fresh mint, minced or ½ teaspoon dried mint

1. Combine all ingredients in blender or food processor until blended. Chill.
2. Serve over fruit salads.

No-Kidding Ketchup

Real ketchup has sugar and salt in it, use this instead.

2 quarts tomatoes, chopped
⅔ cup apple cider vinegar
2 tablespoons honey
2 cloves garlic, freshly minced
　ground black pepper to taste
1 teaspoon basil and/or oregano

1 teaspoon mace
½ to 1 teaspoon dry mustard
1 teaspoon celery seeds
¼ teaspoon sea salt
¼ teaspoon cayenne pepper
1 tablespoon arrowroot

1. In large saucepan, slowly simmer tomatoes over low heat, stirring occasionally. Cook until tomatoes are soft.
2. Push tomatoes through a fine-mesh sieve until only pulp and seeds remain.
3. Add all remaining ingredients, except arrowroot, to strained tomatoes. Return to saucepan, simmer for 30 minutes.
4. If mixture is not thick enough, combine arrowroot with 2 tablespoons water. Stir into tomato mixture and simmer 5 more minutes.
5. Cool before storing in airtight jar.

Mock Sour Cream

On a baked potato I'll take a dab of the real thing, but don't forget this recipe for meals that need some dressing up.

⅔ cup plain low-fat yogurt
⅓ cup low-fat cottage cheese

squeeze of lemon juice

Mix all ingredients in blender until smooth. Chill.

Mustard Dressing

Try this on everything. (Except rice krispies.)

2 tablespoons lemon juice
1 tablespoon Dijon mustard
½ cup olive oil

dash salt
pepper to taste

1. Combine lemon juice and mustard in blender.
2. Add olive oil in constant stream. Blend until creamy. Adjust seasonings.

Poppy Seed Dressing

My way of outdoing the Neiman-Marcus specialty.

2 tablespoons Dijon mustard
1 cup oil
⅓ to ½ cup red wine vinegar

2 tablespoons honey
2 tablespoons poppy seeds
¼ cup grated red onion

1. Combine mustard, oil, vinegar, and honey in blender.
2. Stir in poppy seeds and onion.

Orange Vinaigrette

Light taste for any time of the year.

⅔ cup oil
½ cup red wine vinegar
2 cloves garlic, minced

juice of 1 orange
zest of 1 orange
1 green onion, sliced thin

1. Combine oil, vinegar, garlic, orange juice, and zest in blender
2. Stir in onion

Roquefort Dressing

Too good for mice!

½ cup Roquefort cheese
½ cup plain low-fat yogurt or
    buttermilk
3 tablespoons red wine vinegar

½ teaspoon white pepper
3 tablespoons olive oil
1 clove garlic, peeled

1. Combine cheese, yogurt (or buttermilk), vinegar, and pepper in blender or food processor until smooth.
2. With blender running, slowly add oil and continue until smooth.
3. Place in airtight jar, add garlic clove, and refrigerate. Remove garlic after 24 hours. Blend well before serving.

Spicy Vinegar Dressing

For a little extra spice in your life.

½ cup red wine vinegar
¼ cup water
2 tablespoons fresh lemon juice
2 tablespoons onion, diced

½ teaspoon each: oregano, tarragon, rosemary, thyme, and paprika
½ clove garlic, minced
fresh pepper to taste

Mix all ingredients. Chill. Mix well before serving.

Tarragon Dressing

Grow your own tarragon for even more flavor.

½ cup oil
⅓ cup of wine vinegar
⅛ teaspoon dry mustard
⅛ teaspoon oregano

⅛ teaspoon garlic powder
¼ teaspoon tarragon
salt and pepper to taste

Combine all ingredients and shake well in covered jar.

Cucumber-and-Yogurt Delight

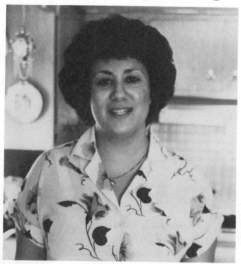

Name: Sammia Haleem
Highest: Close to 200
Now: 159
Goal: 140

My name is Sammia, and my life has changed a lot lately. I've been heavy and tried all the diets, but I never stayed on one before. Now I go to stores and try on new things, and it feels really good. I don't feel stupid anymore. Friends I graduated high school with still say to me, "You look so different. Did you fix your hair a new way?" Well, I did fix my hair, but I fixed everything else too. When I lost all the weight, it all came together for me. I watch Richard every day, and I exercise with the show morning and night and on my own during the day. I'm real happy with my new self.

Ingredients

Serves Two

1 teaspoon lemon juice
2 tablespoons dried, crushed mint leaves
3 tablespoons parsley, chopped
1 small clove garlic, crushed

2 cups plain low-fat yogurt
2 medium cucumbers, sliced or chopped
fresh mint leaves

1. Combine lemon juice, mint, parsley, garlic, and yogurt. Blend well.
2. Stir in cucumber. Refrigerate at least one hour. Garnish with fresh mint.

Overnight Salad

Make it today, enjoy it tomorrow.

Serves Two or Three

Marinade:

½ cup red wine vinegar
⅓ cup oil
¼ cup onion, chopped
1 clove garlic, minced
½ teaspoon honey

½ teaspoon basil
½ teaspoon oregano
¼ teaspoon salt
¼ teaspoon pepper

Vegetables:

1 cup fresh mushrooms, quartered
1 cup celery, sliced
1 cup carrots, sliced
1 cup broccoli florets

1 cup cauliflower, cut into bite-size chunks
½ cup pitted ripe olives, halved
1 ounce pimiento, sliced (optional)

1. In small saucepan, combine the vinegar, oil, honey, onion, basil, garlic, oregano, salt, and pepper. Bring to boil. Simmer 10 minutes.
2. In large plastic bag, combine vegetables and pour hot marinade over them, shake to coat.
3. Place in covered bowl and chill overnight, turning several times.
4. Drain vegetables before serving.

From the kitchen of Paula Lewis

Special Tuna Salad

Richard only wants tuna with good taste, like this one.

Serves Two

1 can tuna, drained and then chilled
2 apples, chopped coarsely
10 stuffed green olives, halved

⅛ teaspoon pepper
3 tablespoons lemon juice
2 tablespoons mayonnaise

1. Mix tuna, apples, olives, pepper, and lemon juice. Add mayonnaise Chill.
2. Serve on bed of lettuce greens.

Seven-Layer Salad

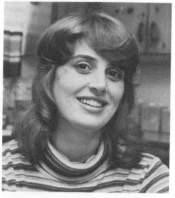

Name: Gail Harper
Highest: 210
Now: 142
Goal: 100

I'm Gail, and this Seven-Layer Salad is one my girl friend and I invented. She started making it, then I started, but I changed it around a little bit. I eat a lot of salads—tuna, three-bean, tomato, onion-and-cucumber—anything. I have to eat a lot of salad to keep the weight off. I bloat otherwise. My husband used to weigh 300 pounds, and he lost 100. That's what gave me the strength to do it. I feel so much better about myself. I'm 32, but my friends say I look 20 or 25 now. I just made up my mind to do it, my husband helped me, and that was it. I'm down from a size 20 pants to a size 14. My friend gave me a top and the size said SMALL. Do you know how proud I feel to wear a small? I was skinny when I got married—95 pounds. But I had a miscarriage and I took birth-control pills and I had 3 children in between, and I got fat. I weighed 210 when I had my last child in January 1981. After that I said I'd lose the weight and never be fat again. I put my mind to it. I have clothes that have been in my closet since I married my husband, and I plan to wear them again!

Ingredients

Serves Four

1 head lettuce or 2 bunches spinach
1¼ cup fresh peas or 1 10-ounce package frozen peas
½ cup water chestnuts, sliced
8 ounces Cheddar or Jack cheese, grated

½ cup unsalted bacon bits or sunflower seeds
4 scallions, finely chopped
2 hard-boiled eggs, sliced

1. Wash lettuce or spinach, tear into bite-size pieces. Steam peas until just tender.
2. Using a large clear salad bowl, layer ingredients in order given. Repeat until all ingredients are used, reserving eggs for the top. Chill.
3. To serve salad, use serving utensils to scoop down through all layers. Each serving should have all the layers.
4. Serve with a vinaigrette dressing on the side.

Fresh Mushroom Salad

A gourmet treat that could be a meal in itself.

Serves Four

1 pound large fresh mushrooms
1 tomato
½ cup scallions, thinly sliced
¼ cup Mock Sour Cream (See p. 161.)
¼ cup olive oil
⅓ cup and 1 tablespoon red wine vinegar

1 tablespoon Gorgonzola or blue cheese
dash of salt
freshly ground pepper
dash garlic powder
¼ teaspoon each marjoram, thyme, dill weed, rosemary
½ teaspoon each basil and sage

1. Wash mushrooms and remove stems. Slice mushrooms and tomatoes as thinly as possible.
2. Combine all other ingredients.
3. Line the outside of a serving platter with the tomato slices. Gently place mushrooms in center of plate. Pour half the dressing over all. Serve remaining dressing on the side.

Wild Watercress Salad

Each bite tastes like springtime (honest!).

Serves Two

3 bunches watercress, in bite-size pieces
1 cup cabbage, shredded
1 large orange, sectioned

½ cup feta cheese, crumbled
⅓ cup onion, sliced in thin rings
¼ cup chopped walnuts (optional)

1. Combine watercress and cabbage. Top with remaining ingredients.
2. Serve with Orange Vinaigrette (See p. 162) or Mustard Dressing (See p. 161).

Rice Salad

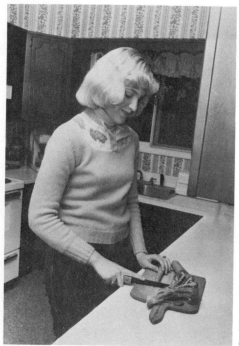

Name: Debbie Mayer
Highest: 169
Now: 145
Goal: 135

Hi. I'm Debbie, and I'm a student in the eighth grade. I'm 5 feet 11 inches and I want to be a model or an actress. I have 10 or 20 more pounds to lose; I want to take off another extra 5 pounds so I never have to worry again. I've lost weight mostly by eating salads—my mom and me eat a lot of salads, my dad likes meat and potatoes— and by exercising. I exercise at least a half hour—and sometimes an hour—every night after dinner.

Ingredients

Serves Six

2 cups long-grain brown rice
2 to 3 tablespoons olive oil
  pepper to taste
1 green bell pepper, diced
1 medium onion, chopped

2 large tomatoes, peeled and chopped
½ cup fresh parsley, chopped
¼ cup fresh basil, chopped
½ cup ripe olives, sliced

1. Cook rice according to package directions. While rice is still warm, toss with oil and pepper.
2. Allow to cool. Add green pepper, onion, tomato, herbs, and olives. Toss gently and chill.
3. Serve in a lettuce-lined bowl.

Dad's Cucumber Salad

This is my dad's favorite, too.

Serves Four

2 cucumbers, thinly sliced
1 sweet Bermuda onion, diced
1/8 teaspoon salt

1/4 teaspoon pepper
1 teaspoon honey
1 cup wine vinegar

1. Combine all ingredients in a 1-quart jar (with a lid). Close and shake well.
2. Chill overnight.

From the kitchen of Shannon Graeser

Chinese Chicken Salad

Great way to use leftovers—and try it with turkey too.

Serves Four to Six

2 cups cooked chicken or turkey, cut up into bite-size pieces
2 medium stalks celery, chopped (about 1 cup)
1 8½-ounce can water chestnuts, drained and sliced

2 green onions, thinly sliced
2 canned pimientos, drained and slivered
1 10-ounce can bamboo shoots, drained and sliced

Dressing:

1/4 cup mayonnaise
1/2 cup plain low-fat yogurt

2 tablespoons tamari
1 tablespoon lemon juice

1. Toss chicken and vegetables together.
2. Stir yogurt, mayonnaise, tamari, and lemon juice together.
3. Chill both mixtures.
4. Serve salad with dressing on the side.

From the kitchen of Barbara Bigelow

Warm Cabbage Salad

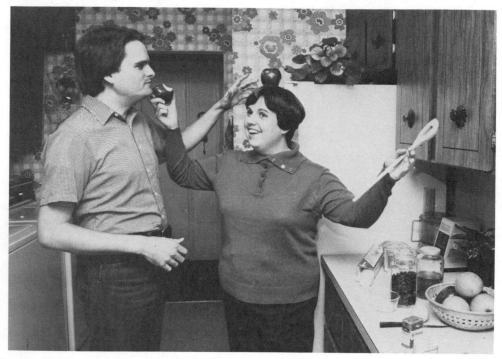

Name: Mary and Robert Graves
Mary's Highest: 275
Robert's Highest: 215
Mary's Now: 191
Robert's Now: 165
Mary's Goal: 115 to 120
Robert's Goal: 145

I'm Mary Graves, and both my husband and I went on the Live-It. I was real heavy, and I thought that when you got to be that heavy, there was no hope for you at all. Then I learned that Richard had lost the weight, and that helped motivate me. I was a heavy child—I had a thyroid problem and all that. Then when I got married, my weight really shot up. That was 7 years ago. I think it was a combination of pressure and candy bars. I was in school and commuting 90 miles, and it was hard to fix regular meals. It was poor stress-management. I began the Live-It in April of 1981, and I lost 77 pounds. I'm so proud of myself. My husband began, too, so we really did it together. My friends have been great, and the nicest part is that people notice that I'm doing what I said I was going to do. They stand back and respect me—and I think I've inspired a few too.

Ingredients

Serves Four

2 cups raw green cabbage, cut into strips
1 cup raw red cabbage, cut into strips
½ cup leeks, sliced and separated into rings
½ cup fresh mushrooms
½ cup zucchini

2 teaspoons sesame oil
1 teaspoon vinegar
2 teaspoons Dijon mustard
caraway seed to taste
freshly ground black pepper, to taste

1. Put sesame oil and vinegar in a nonstick skillet. When hot, add cabbage, zucchini, leeks, and mushrooms, and stir well.
2. Add mustard, caraway seed, and pepper, and stir until vegetables are *al dente*.

Vegetable Salad

Easy to make and great for your figure.

Serves Four to Six

1 head cauliflower, cut into florets
1 pound fresh mushrooms, sliced
1 zucchini, sliced

1 head broccoli, cut into florets
1 small onion, chopped
1 pepper or 6 slices pimientos

Combine all vegetables and garnish with pimientos. Serve with Tarragon Dressing (See page 163).

From the kitchen of Sandy Torres

Delightful Taco Salad Bar

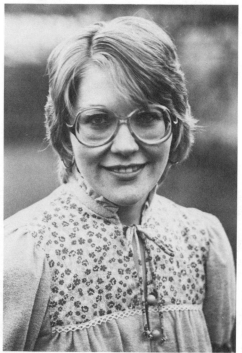

Name: Joanne Jones
Highest: 195
Now: 125
Goal: to stay 125

Hi, I'm Joanne. I was never overweight in my childhood, but in 1977 when I became pregnant with my daughter, Misty, I thought "Ah-ha, now I can eat anything." But it doesn't work that way. I weighed 135 when I got pregnant, and I went into the hospital to have Misty weighing 190. She weighed only 7 pounds 6 ounces, so I left the hospital about 185. I lost weight and got down to 145, then I became pregnant again with my son, Travis. I really watched it that time, so I only gained up to 180. But then after he was born, I went up to 195. Then I thought, "This is enough." A lot of things clicked, and I made a bet with a girl friend on a ten-pound loss. I wasn't going to let her win that bet. I saw Richard on television, and he inspired me. So I won that bet, started watching Richard, cut down on salt, began to exercise 6 times a day (15 minutes at a time) and the pounds started coming off. I had to cut out all goodies. I don't even have a bite, because then I'd want the whole thing. I like to eat salads, and that's helped me a lot. My husband used to call me Love Steamer because I was bigger than the Love Boat, but now he's very proud and he doesn't call me Love Steamer anymore.

Ingredients

Great for a Party

lettuce, any type or a mixture of different
  ones
grated carrots
chopped celery
chopped bell peppers
chopped onions
cubed zucchini
grated cheese
sliced mushrooms

cherry tomatoes or cubed tomatoes
cubed avocado
chopped olives
kidney beans, cooked
crushed taco or tortilla chips—salt-free,
  no preservatives
ground chicken or turkey, browned and
  kept warm on warming tray.
salsa

Serve everything in separate containers. Guests make their own taco salad according to their own tastes.

Tomato Yogurt Salad

Easy, cool and delicious!

Serves Two

2 tomatoes
1 cucumber, thinly sliced
1 stalk celery, chopped
¼ cup yogurt

1 teaspoon creamed horseradish
½ teaspoon honey
  freshly ground pepper to taste
1 green onion, chopped

1. Using a small sharp knife, cut a continuous spiral of peel from each tomato. Turn peel inside out and coil to resemble a rose.
2. Dice remainder of tomato. Combine with remaining ingredients except green onion.
3. Serve in a bed of salad greens. Sprinkle green onion over top of salad. Garnish with tomato roses.

From the kitchen of Pamela Fisher

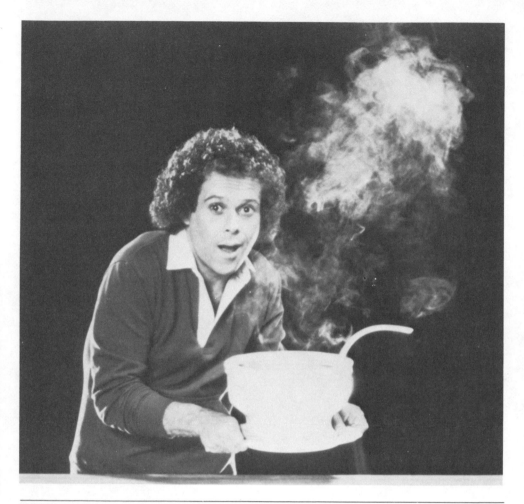

SOUPS ON

I grew up eating soups from red-and-white cans and loving them. Soup and sandwich was my favorite lunch. I put the sandwich directly into the bowl of soup. This was great fun because (a) you could pretend that the sandwich was a buried treasure and (b) you could watch the soup raise up to the top of the bowl while you prayed that it wouldn't go over the edge and spill on the table.

Of course, I wouldn't begin to touch the soup if it weren't smothered in an entire box of crumbled saltines. None of the plain crackers would do. It had to be the kind with the salt crystals on them. And I had to crumble them myself, because I had a very special method. I developed this method over the years while waiting for the soup to cool.

You see, one of my biggest complaints

about soup was that you had to wait all that time for it to boil and then you had to wait again for it to cool off enough so you could eat it. It made little sense to me. But if you spent the waiting minutes crumbling crackers in systematic fashion, the time went more happily.

My parents were both excellent cooks, so we had a lot of homemade soups. Mother bought a huge stockpot—about twenty-five gallons big—at a restaurant supply store and made batches of soup for the freezer in individual portions, first in Tupperware containers and later in Seal-A-Meal plastics so you could just warm them up in hot water. Mother's soups were a meal—we didn't eat them as a meal, we considered them a first course, but that's how I got to weigh 268 pounds—and they were wonderful. So in no time at all I began experimenting with my own soup recipes.

Cream of marshmallow was my least successful—have you ever seen what the bottom of the pan looks like after you've melted all those marshmallows in condensed milk and brandy? I also made my own gumbos. Gumbo was very popular in New Orleans, and everyone else's gumbo really upset me. It seemed that every time I put my face into the food, someone or something was either staring up at me or about to claw me to death. So I made my own gumbo with rubber animals from the dime store. I used dinosaurs, plastic lizards, and all that kind of stuff to make a very successful gumbo. You just had to remember not to eat the animals. But at least I never killed anything. And I didn't have to keep thinking about *Jaws*.

I think everyone has fond memories of soup. It must be because soup is one of the most basic foods ever invented. In fact, long before there were crockpots, microwaves, and designer cookware, there was just one big cast-iron pot (this was after fire but before stainless) that hung from a tripod over a fire and served up all the family meals—porridge in the morning and soup at night. (You had corn tack for lunch, which you ate on the road westward ho or in the fields, which you were hoe hoe hoeing.) Anyway, if the soup had an abundance of meat or chicken in it, it was called stew. More than likely it had in it whatever was available, boiled in water with a touch of salt and some seasonings. When one wanted to look really rich, a little flour or some cream was added to the broth to thicken it and the neighbors were duly impressed. It doesn't make any sense that the more we messed up the soup with fattening ingredients, the more our neighbors respected us, but that's the way it was then. Lean was mean and cream was cream.

Naturally enough, as we became more and more civilized, our eating habits became less civilized. Soups stopped being served as the main meal and became first courses, palate cleansers, or even desserts. Or—the ultimate insult—soups were added to the menu in haste when a few extra heads showed up for dinner and there wasn't enough food: a soup was added to fill up the guests so they didn't notice the scarcity of victuals.

Soup didn't get to be—you should excuse the expression—hot again until recently. Then some soup company decided that there were male and female soups. Female soups were light and airy. Male soups were macho. And so the meal-in-a-can-of-soup idea was reborn. And people took to it as if it were a brand-new idea.

There was only one problem: to keep the meal in the can from turning black, a ton of preservatives, chemicals, flavor-enhancers, and thickeners had to be added to the already overcooked vegetables and the reconstituted meat or chicken bitlets. But some people really do like to eat chemicals.

As the soup revolution went on, packaged soups in individual packets became popular. Soup as a snack was thought to be better for you than milk and cookies. This sounds right, but if you're eating a soup that's all chemicals, you may be dead wrong. So here are a few soup tips to keep in mind when you're making your choices:

Read labels on cans and packages. There are some good ones on the market, but you have to be careful. Soups can be like salad dressings, so watch out.

Soup makes a good meal, especially in the evening, because it's light.

If your soup has pasta in it, don't eat bread.

Soup is a good meal to order in a restaurant if the regular entrées look too rich for your food plan.

Soups can be inexpensive to make because you can make them with leftovers.

Soups freeze well.

Homemade soups are better than canned or packaged soups.

Soups are great for people who work—put the ingredients in a crockpot before you leave for work and come home to a hot and nutritious meal.

Before you buy expensive packaged soups, look at the dehydrated goods on the same shelf and combine them with fresh ingredients for a homemade soup.

Avoid cream-, milk-, or sour cream–based recipes. A touch of sherry is okay though.

If you're eating soup and salad together as a meal, have a cup of soup and half a salad.

Eat bread with your soup only if you've not had bread during the day.

If you add bread to the soup, that counts as bread. Do not add salt-laden crackers or packaged goodies that swim in the broth and then swim directly to your hips.

Soup making is the best way to make a little bit of food go a long way.

Making soup can relieve stress.

CREAMY DREAMY SOUPS

One of the things I hate the most about dingdong diets is that they tell you to make all kinds of crazy substitutions. I was reading a magazine once and—I swear this is true—I saw a recipe (and a picture to back it up, in glorious Koda-chrome) for fake linguine and clams. The clams were real clams, but the linguine was shredded celery stalks. Well, I about wet my pants. I've been very careful with all my recipes to make sure that the in-gredients we ask you to use as substitu-tions are not ridiculous.

So it makes perfect sense for me to tell you to cut out creamy and milky soups. Or you can also do what I do. Use low-fat or skim milk and then throw in a tad of nonfat powdered milk as thickener. This way you get all the joys of creamy soups with few of the calories. Or lumps.

THE MEDICAL DICTIONARY OF SOUP

Mother was right about chicken soup. It does cure colds. It does mend broken hearts. It warms, it comforts, it heals, it soothes. And this isn't just speculation. Scientists have been testing mom's theo-ries and have proved her right (was there ever any doubt?)—chicken soup can make you well again.

So with this in mind, we've hired a few mad scientists to begin testing the other soups readily available to mankind to see what scientific discoveries can be made.

Turkey Soup: Nope, it doesn't turn you into a turkey. Don't get smart with me. Turkey soup happens to help insomnia. Honest. It has tryptophan in it, and that means a nice quiet rest for your nerves, and then it's sandman time.

Consommé: A clear or brownish clear soup served hot or jellied at weddings to celebrate the union of the bride and groom. In some cultures it is believed that the cold consommé—or the jellied version—portends a longer-lasting union, or a marriage that gels.

Onion Soup: Another wedding soup, which was once called union soup. This one is known for its fertility powers.

Vichyssoise, A cold potato soup known to cure the French Disease.

Beef and Barley Soup: Recently discov-ered to cure acne, blackheads, pimples, and eczema in teeners.

Wonton Soup: Cures many strains of Asian flu. Also helpful in treatment of nymphomaniacs.

Cream of Rice: Fights humidity in southern regions and prevents hair from frizzing.

Cream of Tomato: Prevents colds be-cause it has a high percentage of vitamin C. Also may cure blindness when com-bined with grated carrot and Parmesan cheese.

Lobster Bisque: Cures itching symp-toms, jock itch, and rashes.

Saint Germain Soup (Pea Soup): Cures urinary and bladder infections.

Gazpacho: Mends ligaments that were torn or stretched while riding among high pampas.

Minestrone: Eliminates minigallstones.

Gumbo: Heals trenchmouth, canker sores, and denture slippage.

Cock-a-Leekie: (Don't giggle. This is a real soup! It's Scottish. So there.) Cock-a-Leekie soup ends impotence in men over forty-three.

Leekie soup ends bedroom problems in men over forty-three.

Macho Gazpacho

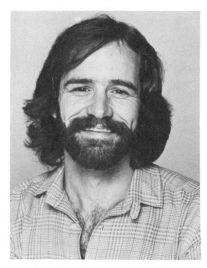

Name: Gregory Loeb
Highest: 183
Now: 140
Goal: To stay there!

My name is Greg Loeb, and I'm hypoglycemic. I was pretty heavy, and it was sort of Catch-22—I ate too many sweets, so I became fat and hypoglycemic and when I had to start watching what I ate, the weight began to come off. What I do is what Richard says. I stay away from sugar and junk foods and I eat a lot of salads. That's why I like this gazpacho recipe—it's salad in soup form. I'm single, so I cook for myself and I end up eating a lot of salads.

Ingredients

Serves Eight to Ten

1 cucumber, seeded
2 green peppers, seeded
6 cups fresh tomatoes
1 small white or yellow onion
1 celery stalk
1½ cups tomato juice
¼ cup red wine vinegar
6 ounces marinated artichoke hearts and oil
1 medium zucchini
1 to 2 ounces pimiento

1 green onion
1 teaspoon freshly ground black pepper
pinch of salt
hot sauce or Tabasco to taste
¼ to ½ teaspoon oregano
¼ teaspoon dried rosemary, crushed
¼ teaspoon dried thyme, crushed
1 teaspoon Italian seasonings (marjoram, savory, sage, basil)
croutons for garnish

1. Reserve ½ cup each coarsely chopped cucumber, green pepper, tomato, white onion, and the croutons.
2. Purée remaining tomatoes in blender. Add all other ingredients and purée. Adjust seasoning and hot sauce to taste. Refrigerate several hours.
3. Serve individual 1-cup portions, to which each guest adds additional accompaniments of the reserved veggies.
4. Garnish with a few croutons.

Carrot Soup

A 40 karat taste treat.

Serves Six

1 onion, chopped	2 cups chicken stock
1 clove garlic, mashed	¼ teaspoon white pepper
3 tablespoons butter	¼ cup nonfat dry powdered milk
4 carrots, grated	½ cup liquid nonfat milk
2 stalks celery, chopped	

1. Sauté onion and garlic in butter. Add carrots and sauté a few more minutes.
2. Add chicken stock and cook until vegetables are cooked soft.
3. Purée soup and add milks (dry milk mixed with whole milk). Return to pot and add pepper.
4. Heat and serve.

Grandma Sophie's Cabbage Soup

This will warm you on a cold damp night. And put on a sweater, darling. Did you practice the piano?

2 pounds brisket or short ribs	2 tablespoons honey
2 soup bones (optional)	pinch salt
1 large onion, diced	pinch pepper
2 cups canned tomatoes, chopped	½ cup seedless grapes (optional)
1 medium head cabbage, shredded	2 quarts water
¼ cup lemon juice	

Bring meat, bones and water to rapid boil. Skim off fat and simmer one hour. Add cabbage and remaining ingredients. Simmer until meat is tender. Taste and correct seasoning.

From the kitchen of Susan Goldstein

Apple Apricot Dream Soup

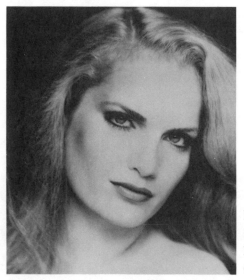

Name: Idrea Lippman
Highest: 252 (when pregnant)
Now: 187
Goal: 140

My name is Idrea and I have some incredible things to tell you. I was one of the few women in this country who like being fat. I've been a large size model for over four years, I'm with Wilhelmina, one of the best model agencies, and people tell me I look great all the time even though I wear a size 20. There's this whole big feminist movement going on now that it's okay to be fat, but I think that 98% of the women who are fat really want to be thin. I've given all this an incredible amount of thought, because I've been having what you can call a life crisis. I actually make a good living from being fat. And I've decided to give it up. I might look good as a size 20 but deep inside I know I'd look better as a size 12.

I've been heavy all my life. I was born fat. I never even tried a lot of diets because they were too much trouble. I like to pig-out. Then I read about Richard and I called him and I went to class. He was really impressive. He's honest and now I do what he says. I've lost 35 pounds. Now I eat sensibly because Richard is motivating me. And I exercise at least three times a week. I just don't feel good when I don't exercise.

I came up with this recipe while I was fooling around in the kitchen. I like foods that are different, that have taste. I'm not the kind who can live on cottage cheese or hard-boiled eggs. I make this cold soup for my family all the time. You can use apple juice or substitute pear nectar or peach, but be sure to get it from the health food store so it has no sugar in it. And you can add a dash of sherry or fruit wine if you want to dress it up a bit.

Ingredients

Serves Eight

3 cups fresh apricots (chopped)
2 cups clear apple juice

1 pint plain yogurt

1. Puree apricot, apple juice in a blender.
2. Put in large bowl. Whisk in yogurt.
3. Cover and refrigerate until cold.
4. Serve sprinkled with wheat germ or granola.

Chicken Zucchini Soup

Why did the chicken cross the road? To have the soup, of course.

Serves Fifteen

2 cups cooked chicken, skinned, boned, and chopped
4 cups zucchini, chopped
4 cups fresh tomatoes, peeled and chopped
1 cup green and red bell peppers, chopped

1 cup celery, chopped
1 cup onion, chopped
1 clove garlic, chopped
$1/4$ teaspoon Vegit or poultry seasoning
10 ounces low-sodium V-8 juice
$1/2$ teaspoon salt
pepper to taste

1. Combine all ingredients except chicken in large saucepan. Simmer on low heat until all vegetables are tender.
2. Purée in batches. Return to saucepan, add chicken and adjust seasoning.
3. Reheat and serve.

From the kitchen of Sandy Owens

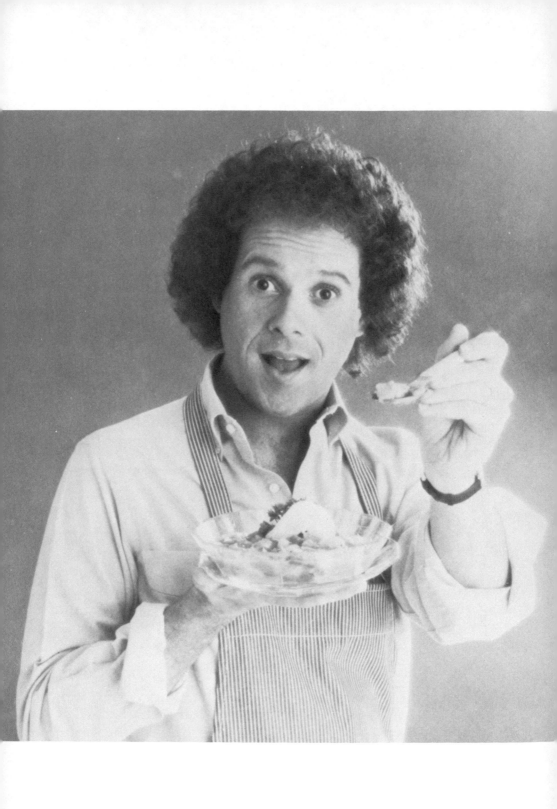

Just Desserts

THE HISTORY OF DESSERT

Are you one of those people who has trouble spelling *dessert* and gets it mixed up with *desert*? It's an easy problem to have. And there's a very good reason why. Because long ago and far away, dessert was invented out in the desert.

Our story goes all the way back to the Creation. We all know what the world looked like in ancient times because we've seen *The Ten Commandments*, right? Well, someplace in the midst of all that sand was a little oasis called the Gar-

den of Eden. (Not to be confused with the Garden of Allah.) The Garden of Eden was a very nice place to grow up in—lots of apple trees, a few pet snakes to play with. It was a bit rural, and there weren't too many neighborhood children to play with, but suburbia hadn't been discovered yet, and there was not much Adam and Eve could do about their plight. So they took to raising Cain—and Abel, too, of course.

The boys never did get along very well, and Eve spent a good bit of her day trying to make things better for them.

Whenever one of them would have a fight with the other, he would invariably come crying into the kitchen and need some tender loving care. Eve spelled TLC the way every mother since has: F-O-O-D.

"Don't worry, sweetheart," Eve would say in her soothing voice, "Mommy will make it better." And mommy served a hot apple-and-grape pie. (They hadn't figured out yet that you had to dry the grapes to get raisins.) Eve was famous for her apple pie—she was known throughout the land for her way with apples, and she also had a knack for the right extra touches. It was she who first thought of adding a touch of cinnamon—she called it Original Cinnamon back then—and came up with the grapes. Rum sauce and Cheddar cheese were just a step away.

It was Eve's contention that a great dessert could take your mind off all your problems and set your entire being into a state of relaxation and satisfaction. These were two states she craved, because we all know how hard it is raising two boys, especially without day-care, neighbors, or Play-Doh. Her method seemed to have worked, and throughout history, the idea of dessert as a cure-all began to develop.

When Cain killed Abel, Mom served apple tarts. When Rome burned, Nero snacked on Mallomars, bringing the cookies closer and closer to his nose so he could smell the chocolate and not the smoke. After Napoleon froze in Russia he returned home to some hot chocolate and an éclair. And we can only suppose that while Hitler sat in his bunker, watching his mad dreams fall to extinction, Eva Braun was baking Black Forest cake.

Things may go better with Coke. But dessert makes them even better.

Being ingrained so deeply in history, the notion that you can live happily without dessert is a hard one to shake. I know. I have the same problems you do. My mommy always told me that a nice hot meal would make me feel better. And the topper to a nice hot meal was a nice dessert.

Dessert, we have all come to believe, is something that we have earned just for not giving in to our problems. Dessert seems to be life's most basic reward.

Now, I ask you, does that make any sense? Should something that can make you fat and sloppy and crazy from sugar and cavities—and even cost you your life—be the beginning and the end of happiness? Of course not. But to many people dessert is what they deserve. Dessert is what they have earned, just by being alive.

So I've got big news for you, America. You'll be a lot more alive when you lose twenty pounds and step into clothes a size smaller.

So reprogram your mind and your body. Forget all about the genetic history you have been carrying with you for two billion years. I'm not advocating banning all desserts. Heaven forbid. I just want you to realize that you can live a perfectly healthy and happy life if you don't have a dessert—let alone two, three, or four desserts—in a day. Save desserts for special occasions. Taste desserts and then leave them on your plate. Cook desserts that are not as bad for you as other desserts. Learn to love yourself enough to say "No, thanks; not today."

THE DESSERT-O-HOLICS QUIZ

Dessert seems to be the downfall of every dieter you've ever met. That's why I like the Live-It so much. You get to have dessert. Not after every meal, mind you. But if you want it—you got it. All you need to do is exercise it off and eat a small portion. Come on, admit it—you didn't plan to go through life craving Toll House cookies but never eating them again, now, did you?

There happen to be sensible ways and not so sensible ways to eat dessert. But before we even get to them, let's find out just how dedicated you are to dessert. Fill in this little questionnaire and we'll see if you're a mere faddist or if you have a sweet tooth that cannot be denied.

1. Maida Heatter is:
a. a solar device that saves energy while keeping your home warm.
b. an author of several fine cookbooks of dessert recipes.
c. a woman who cleans and eats leftovers without heating them up.

2. *Crème Fraîche* is:
a. fresh cream for your coffee.
b. a pudding served in a heart-shaped porcelain dish.
c. a sour cream–like mixture, great with strawberries.

3. The only dessert worth eating is:
a. chocolate.
b. chocolate.
c. chocolate.

4. Soufflé is:
a. a see-through fabric imported from Hong Kong and used in evening gowns.
b. a dessert made of eggs, air, and hopefully chocolate or Grand Marnier.
c. a hairstyle popular just before the bouffant.

5. Toll House cookies are:
a. made by gnomes and sold under a bridge.
b. given away at toll stations on state-funded highways.
c. Nestlé's recipe for the world's best chocolate chip cookies.

6. Le Nôtre is:
a. a famous church in Paris.
b. a famous patisserie in Paris.
c. a famous college football team.

7. A bain-marie is:
a. a bath for a dirty French girl named Mary.
b. a type of double boiler for baking.
c. an exotic French werewolf curse.

8. Yeast is:
a. a brewer's secret ingredient.
b. granulated or cubed for baking.
c. the opposite direction from ywest.

9. Gugelhupf is:
a. a type of dessert mold.
b. a German youth movement.
c. a noodle pudding.

10. *Pain au chocolat* is:
a. the pain you get from living without chocolate.
b. a French pastry filled with chocolate.
c. acne from too much chocolate.

11. Meringue is:
a. a wild Spanish dance.
b. a tomato sauce for rice, shrimp, or chicken.
c. beaten and baked egg whites, usually atop desserts and pies.

12. *Gâteau* is French for:
a. Cat.
b. Boat.
c. Cake.

13. Crepes suzettes are:
a. thin pancakes with orange liqueur sauce.
b. French slang for what a baby does in his diapers.
c. a chain of restaurants serving fast-food crepes.

14. Yorkshire pudding is:
a. an eggy pancake that has nothing whatsoever to do with dessert.
b. a pudding served with heavy cream and raisins.
c. a nickname for the kind of terrier indigenous to that region of England.

15. A Norwegian omelet is:
a. a flat egg dish topped with sardines and onions.
b. a backpack that folds in half that originated in Scandinavia.
c. another name for Baked Alaska.

16. A tart is:
a. a girl of loose reputation.
b. a dessert topped with fruit.
c. a version of a sacher torte.

17. A coupe is:
a. a jazzy sports car.
b. a dessert with ice cream.
c. an attempt to overthrow a government.

18. Glacé is:
a. Italian dessert ice.
b. Glazed fruit topping on coffee cakes.
c. An expert at repairing broken windows.

19. Puff pastry is:
a. A light airy pastry made from many layers of dough that forms the basis of French pastries such as éclairs.
b. the kind of pastry preferred by dragons.
c. a fluffy pastry reminiscent of a powder puff.

20. I get confused when spelling *dessert* and *desert:*
a. some of the time.
b. none of the time.
c. all of the time.

Use this chart to score your test:

1. a. 1 pt.		b. 3 pts.		c. 2 pts.
2. a. 1 pt.		b. 2 pts.		c. 3 pts.
3. a. 3 pts.		b. 3 pts.		c. 3 pts.
4. a. 1 pt.		b. 3 pts.		c. 2 pts.
5. a. 2 pts.		b. 1 pt.		c. 3 pts.
6. a. 1 pt.		b. 3 pts.		c. 2 pts.
7. a. 2 pts.		b. 3 pts.		c. 1 pt.
8. a. 2 pts.		b. 3 pts.		c. 1 pt.

9. a. 3 pts.	b. 1 pt.	c. 2 pts.
10. a. 1 pt.	b. 3 pts.	c. 2 pts.
11. a. 1 pt.	b. 2 pts.	c. 3 pts.
12. a. 1 pt.	b. 2 pts.	c. 3 pts.
13. a. 3 pts.	b. 1 pt.	c. 2 pts.
14. a. 3 pts.	b. 2 pts.	c. 1 pt.
15. a. 1 pt.	b. 2 pts.	c. 3 pts.
16. a. 1 pt.	b. 3 pts.	c. 2 pts.
17. a. 1 pt.	b. 3 pts.	c. 2 pts.
18. a. 3 pts.	b. 3 pts.	c. 1 pt.
19. a. 3 pt.	b. 2 pts.	c. 1 pt.
20. a. 2 pts.	b. 3 pts.	c. 1 pt.

TOTAL Your Score

If your score is 55–60

Oh, my goodness! Nothing gets by you, does it? You probably studied dessertery at Cordon Bleu and have been memorizing cookbooks since you were seven. Tell me, c'mon, whisper in my ear: Is there any dessert you haven't tried? Is there one you don't like?

If your score is 54–45

You have an extremely healthy—or should I say unhealthy—knowledge of desserts. I daresay someone gave you cooking lessons for Christmas one year, and you just can't stop taking those classes when you see the word *chocolate* mentioned in the brochure. Chances are you even opened to this chapter first, just to check it out before you bought the book. Sorry there aren't any color pictures, I know you're disappointed.

If your score is 44–35

You're my kind of person. You got about half the answers right, but there were a lot of technical French terms you didn't know. It doesn't mean you don't like dessert, you just like what you know and don't go in for highfalutin stuff. You're the chocolate-cake-and-a-glass-of-milk-at-bedtime type, I know it.

If your score is 34–24

That's okay, don't be embarrassed by this answer. We all know you've been in a satellite orbiting the Earth for the past fifty-two years and haven't quite caught up with what's going on with the rest of us. Your answers were very good; they just weren't right for the category of desserts. But that's okay with me. You're probably thin as a potato chip and have no cravings for sugar whatsoever.

If your score is below 24

Are you sure you're alive? Check into the nearest hospital for a blood test immediately. Then call me and explain how you possibly got a score this low. But congratulations, you're probably a thin person.

DESSERT TRAPS AND HOW TO AVOID THEM

Dessert Trap #1: You are hunched over your desk studying a computer printout that makes your eyes water and your head pound. You skipped breakfast because you woke up late. You must finish this printout and analyze it before lunch because there's a meeting with your boss at two and you have a lunch meeting with the client prior to that. Someone from down the hall sticks his head in your office and announces, "There's a coffee cake Janet brought in today, want some?" or "It's Adele's birthday today. Have you had any cake yet?" You know that a break for some cake and a good hot cup of coffee will make you work much better. You did skip breakfast. You are hungry. You need it to survive. You deserve it for working so hard.

Solution: Eat breakfast next time, silly. We've told you about that a million times. And we're skipping coffee breaks now, remember? Say "No, thank you" and close your office door.

Dessert Trap #2: You've just eaten one of the best meals of your life in a very fancy restaurant. You are so stuffed that you have to unbutton your shirt in order to breathe. The dessert cart rolls around. Everyone at the table ooohs and aaaahs. You suggest sharing a dessert with someone else, knowing full well you have no right eating dessert. The other person says no, she wants her own dessert. You get a bowl of chocolate mousse topped with whipped cream. Even though you thought you'd only have a few bites, you have just eaten the entire portion and licked the inside of the bowl with your tongue.

Solution: Eat less at lunch and don't finish the dessert. If you had paced yourself properly, you would have been able to eat a little of each course and been satisfied without being bloated, and you still could have had a taste of dessert. Instead, you pigged out. What ever happened to common sense and discipline anyway?

Dessert Trap #3: You go to someone's house—someone you don't know that well but would like to know better—and they offer you dessert. You want to explain that you've cut out desserts but are afraid of being rude. You take the dessert and just eat a bite or two to be polite. But then the hostess eyes your plate suspiciously and asks if you didn't like her cooking. You finish everything on the plate and leave with a tinfoil CARE package for your refrigerator.

Solution: Don't accept dessert in the first place. Smile and say "No, thank you." Try it, you may get used to it. Remember, there will always be dessert. You have to learn how to live with it.

A WORD ABOUT HEALTHFUL DESSERTS

It's been a relatively well-known fact over the past fifty, maybe even a hundred, years, that desserts are fattening. They are wonderful, but they are fattening. This didn't pose a big problem to many cultures or strata of society—Victorians, for example, happened to like their women a little on the chunky side, and first-generation Americans liked to produce fat children because it showed the world how rich they were—after all, they were no longer starving. But, well, when thin became "in," dessert became dangerous.

So Madison Avenue set to finding new ways to make us believe that we could eat dessert without gaining weight. In the late 1950s ice milk became very popular. Ice milk is a substitute for ice cream only in that it has a higher water content and lower milk and butterfat content than ice cream. It doesn't taste like ice cream, but it doesn't taste bad. In fact, of all the desserts I've sampled—especially the ones that claim to be "dietetic"—ice milk holds up as one of the best.

Shortly thereafter you may have noticed a whole special area in your grocery store—it's usually the other side of the shelf that has all the Manischewitz products—come into being: the "dietetic foods" area. All kinds of newfangled desserts emerged: cookies and cakes that weren't supposed to be fattening, gelatins and puddings that claimed to have only a handful of calories, and all kinds of fake milk shake drinks. These foods were supposed to satisfy your craving for dessert while not polluting your body with excess calories. What the manufacturers failed to mention is that they were polluting your body with chemicals instead.

And you all know how I feel about chemicals. I'm the one who told you to use real butter instead of margarine, remember? I do not like synthetic anything, and I am highly suspicious of foods that are made of the same things that polyester is made of.

I must not have been the only one to have been wary, because shortly thereafter, by the late 1960s, the Healthful Revolution had taken over. The byword of the health-food nuts became *carrot cake.* Suddenly chocolate cake was out and carrot cake was in. Or banana nut or alfalfa raisin or zucchini cinnamon. Well,

let me tell you about carrot cake. It may look healthful. It may come in a whole-earth kind of simple brown wrapper that says NO CHEMICALS on it. It may be made of God's own carrots, raisins, and honey. But it is still fattening. About the smallest ingredient in carrot cake is carrots. And then once you bake the cake, you have to frost it: That cream cheese icing is mixed with sugar and then topped with a marzipan orange carrot with green leaves. Cute? Very. Fattening? You betcha.

Along with the natural foods kick came the yogurt kick. People suddenly got the great idea that ice cream was fattening but frozen yogurt wasn't. They flocked in herds to yogurt stands and asked for carob sprinkles instead of jimmies on top of their strawberry-flavored frozen yogurt in the whole wheat sugar cone. They bought push-up snacks of flavored frozen yogurt for their children, weaning them off Fudgsicles for something that was not only healthful but not fattening. They all but boycotted the baked goods department of the grocery store as they chained their bikes to the Yoplait bikestand out front and stocked up on any of the six dozen new flavors of yogurt. And when the news was broadcast, no one wanted to listen: Yogurt may have just as many calories as ice cream. Plain old yogurt does not. Flavored yogurt may.

So what's a person to do?

Eat dessert. Avoid desserts that promise you they aren't fattening. They're lying to you. Avoid appetite-suppressing foods that are supposed to taste like cookies or breakfast bars but don't. Eat real old-fashioned desserts. But do it in moderation.

WHEN TO EAT DESSERT

Dessert is a sacred thing and should be treated as a special experience for the right occasions in your life. Since the Live-It is not one of those so rigid diets that you have to walk around with a piece of paper telling you what to eat each day, I cannot really tell you to follow this list. But keep it in mind. It's my own personal list of when and when not to indulge and it makes sure I don't overindulge.

When to eat dessert:
- On your birthday
- At your wedding
- At the wedding of someone you love
- At your child's birthday party
- After lunch
- When you are celebrating a happy occasion

When not to eat dessert:
- At an office birthday party
- At a wedding for someone you barely know
- At all the other children's birthday parties you go to with your child
- After dinner
- When you are sad or depressed

REMEMBER: Just because everyone around you may be eating dessert, doesn't mean you have to join in. You're not a lemming. (Don't know what a lemming is? I didn't either until I read a children's book. It seems that these little buggers live and die by playing follow the leader. If the leader goes off a cliff, so do all the other lemmings.) Think for yourself! And when you do take dessert, you don't have to finish it. And if you do finish it, you certainly don't need another piece.

Stuffed Apples

A new twist on baked apples that your family will love.

Serves Six

6 apples	¼ teaspoon cinnamon
¾ cup mixture of walnuts, raisins, and chopped dried apricots	⅛ teaspoon nutmeg
	¾ cup water
2 tablespoons honey	3 tablespoons butter

1. Core a 1- to 1½-inch hole from center of apple, leaving bottom intact.
2. Mix nut mixture with 1 tablespoon honey and spices. Fill apples with mixture.
3. Place in baking dish, dot each apple with ½ teaspoon butter.
4. Mix ¾ cup water with 1 tablespoon honey, dot with butter, and place in oven. Pour into baking dish.
5. Bake in 300°F oven for 1 hour, basting every few minutes.

Orange Cream Puffs

Just don't eat the whole batch yourself!

Serves Eighteen

Cream Puffs:

⅓ cup margarine	1 cup flour, sifted
½ cup water	4 eggs
½ teaspoon salt	

Filling:

6 ounces frozen unsweetened orange juice, defrosted	15 ounces part-skim ricotta cheese
	⅛ teaspoon salt

1. Heat margarine with water until mixture boils. Reduce heat to low and add salt and flour. Stir until mixture leaves the sides of the pan and is in a smooth, compact ball.
2. Remove from pan and place in a mixing bowl. Add eggs, one at a time. Beat well until smooth and shiny.
3. Drop mixture by spoonfuls, 3 inches apart, on ungreased cookie sheet. Bake in preheated 350°F oven for 30 minutes. Turn oven off and remove cookie sheet.
4. Make a slit in the top of each puff, then return to oven for 10 more minutes. Slice a thin layer from the top of each puff.
5. Combine filling ingredients and beat until smooth. Spoon into cream puffs.

Bread Pudding

As old fashioned as merrie olde England but not as fattening.

Serves Six

2 eggs
2 tablespoons honey
1 teaspoon vanilla
 cinnamon
2 cups milk, scalded

3 slices whole grain bread, toasted,
 lightly buttered, and cut into cubes
¼ cup raisins
 nutmeg

1. In bowl, beat eggs, honey, vanilla, and cinnamon. Slowly add scalded milk.
2. Put bread and raisins in 1½ quart casserole dish. Pour milk mixture over and sprinkle with additional cinnamon and nutmeg. Stand casserole in large pan with 1 inch of water.
3. Bake in 325°F oven for 1 hour.

Frozen Fruit Salad (Popsticks*)

A delicious snack for you or the kids.

Serves Ten

2 fresh peaches
1 cup fresh strawberries
1 cup fresh cherries, pitted
1 8-ounce can crushed pineapple
½ cup fresh blueberries
1¼ cups plain low-fat yogurt
¾ cup low-fat cottage cheese

4 tablespoons honey
2 tablespoons lemon juice
4 tablespoons frozen orange juice
 concentrate
⅛ teaspoon salt
¼ teaspoon vanilla extract

1. Poach peaches in boiling water for 1 minute. Peel and cut into thin wedges.
2. Hull strawberries and slice thinly. Cut pitted cherries in half. Drain pineapple well, reserving juice. Rinse and clean blueberries.
3. In blender, combine yogurt, cottage cheese, honey, lemon juice, orange juice, salt, vanilla, and reserved pineapple juice.
4. Layer fruits in a 2-quart bowl. Pour yogurt mixture over fruits. Freeze until firm. Allow to thaw slightly before serving. Slice in 1-inch wedges.
 *To make Popsticks, divide fruit into 10 6-ounce paper cups. Pour yogurt mixture over the fruit. Place wooden sticks or a plastic spoon in the center of each cup. Freeze until firm.

Cheeseless Cheesecake

I dare you to miss the cheese.

Serving Size: One Two-inch slice

½ cup granola
½ cup boiling water
2 packages unflavored gelatin
20 ounces crushed pineapple
1⅓ cup dry powdered low-fat milk
3 teaspoons vanilla extract
1 tablespoon orange juice concentrate

2 teaspoons lemon juice
1 ripe banana
1 teaspoon each orange and lemon
  rind, grated
strawberries
cinnamon

1. Line the bottom of an 8-inch or 9-inch pie plate with granola. Sprinkle gelatin over water. Let stand 2 minutes.
2. Add water, pineapple, dry milk, vanilla, orange juice, lemon juice, and banana to blender or food processor. Blend until smooth and fluffy.
3. Stir in grated rind. Turn onto pie plate. Chill until firm. Garnish with strawberries and cinnamon. Cut into 2-inch slices.

From the kitchen of Karol DiCiccio

Peach Cobbler

Southern down home goodness that beats Sara Lee.

Serves Four to Six

4 cups sliced fresh peaches
2 tablespoons honey
1 egg, well beaten
1 tablespoon tapioca granules
½ teaspoon cinnamon
½ teaspoon vanilla extract

1 cup whole wheat pastry flour
1 teaspoon soda
1 tablespoon butter
⅓ cup buttermilk
¼ cup milk

1. Combine peaches, honey, egg, tapioca, cinnamon, and vanilla.
2. Preheat oven to 425°F. Grease a 9-inch round baking dish.
3. Spread peach mixture evenly on bottom of baking dish.
4. Mix flour, soda, butter, milk, and buttermilk into dough. Roll dough to ¼-inch thickness. Prick dough with fork and place loosely over peaches. Bake 20 to 30 minutes.
   Serve with fresh puréed peaches for topping.

The Lemoniest Meringue Pie

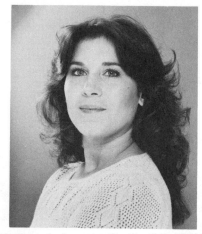

Name: Anita Rena Nuñez
Highest: 144
Now: 121
Goal: 118

My name is Anita, and I had a weight problem when I was eleven years old. I was just chubby—they called it baby fat back then. Then when I was 15, I was determined to get thin, so I went on one of those crazy diets where you eat 9 eggs a day and nothing else. I stayed thin till I was about 18 and went away to college. I didn't have much money and I didn't have a regular schedule and I ate a lot of garbage. I was studying nutrition—but I kept eating garbage and gaining weight. I ate bread and rice, peanut butter, and bread and rice, and macaroni and cheese and bread and rice and peanut butter, and well, you get the idea. I went to college weighing 118 and left weighing 144. Then I read the Live-It, and I decided it was perfect for me because I wanted a life plan not a diet. I went a little slower than Richard says; my portions weren't as small, so it took me a year to lose 20 pounds. And I dance for 2 hours at least 3 times a week—sometimes 5 times. I stopped eating meat, I stopped snacks, and I always keep an eye on my intake.

Ingredients

Serves Twelve

Crust:

1¼ cup whole wheat pastry flour
 ¼ teaspoon baking soda
 ¼ teaspoon salt
 5 tablespoons butter

1 egg
1 tablespoon lemon juice
1 tablespoon water

Filling and Meringue:

⅔ cup honey
⅓ cup arrowroot
tiny pinch of salt
1¼ cup boiling water
½ cup lemon juice

1 tablespoon grated lemon peel
5 eggs, separated
1 tablespoon honey
1 teaspoon lemon juice
1 teaspoon vanilla extract

1. In mixing bowl, combine flour, soda, and salt. Cut butter into flour mixture until pieces are about the size of peas.
2. Combine egg, lemon juice, and water. Slowly blend into flour mixture, being careful not to overmix.
3. Roll out dough to fit a 9-inch pie pan. Press dough in pan, then press fork around edges of dough.
4. In top of double boiler, combine honey, arrowroot, and salt. Add boiling water and cook over medium heat until mixture comes to a boil, making sure that water does not touch bottom of top boiler.
5. Slowly add ½ cup lemon juice, lemon peel, and egg yolks. Cook about 10 to 12 minutes, stirring constantly, until mixture thickens. Remove from heat.
6. Beat egg whites until frothy. Slowly add the teaspoon of lemon juice and continue beating until *soft* peaks form. Add honey and vanilla, and continue beating until *stiff* peaks form.
7. When filling comes to room temperature, place in baked pastry shell. Top with meringue.
8. Bake in preheated 400°F oven 6 to 8 minutes, or until meringue is golden brown.

Baked Pineapple

Don't read the ingredients first, just make it, you'll be surprised.

Serves Four

2 cups pineapple chunks
1 cup grated Cheddar cheese
¾ cup pineapple juice
2 tablespoons honey

½ teaspoon vanilla
1 tablespoon whole wheat flour
1 cup whole wheat bread crumbs
1½ tablespoons butter

1. Mix pineapple and cheese in 2-quart casserole.
2. Mix juice, honey, vanilla, and flour and cook until it thickens. Pour over pineapple and cheese.
3. Top with bread crumbs and dot with butter. Bake in 350° F oven for 25 to 30 minutes, or until bubbly.

Zucchini Carrot Cake

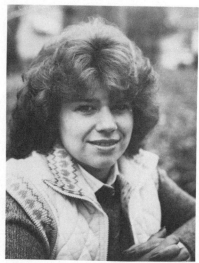

Name: Liz Hoegg
Highest: 260+
Now: 160
Goal: 145

I'm Liz, and believe me, I owe it all to the Live-It. I've been on millions of diets, I've tried all kinds of things, but when I saw Richard on Phil Donahue, he really did something to me. I bought *Never-Say-Diet* that same day, and I began in right away. I work in a mall, and you wouldn't believe what happens. People I don't even know come up to me and tell me how good I look and ask me why I didn't take the weight off a long time ago. My husband loves the new me. My whole life has changed. I exercise at home 2 times a day and I take a jazz class once a week. In addition to managing this photo shop I'm branching out to begin business as a photographer. Everything is working out great now.

Ingredients

Serving Size: One-inch Slice

2 eggs
½ cup honey
1½ cups whole wheat flour
½ cup oil
1 teaspoon baking powder
1 teaspoon baking soda
2 teaspoons cinnamon

1 teaspoon vanilla extract
½ teaspoon sea salt
1 cup carrot, grated
1½ cup zucchini, grated
½ cup crushed pineapple, drained
½ cup chopped nuts (preferably walnuts)

1. Beat eggs with honey until frothy. Gradually beat in oil. Add dry ingredients. Beat at high speed for 4 minutes.
2. Stir in carrot, zucchini, pineapple, and nuts. Pour into lightly greased 9-inch baking pan.
3. Bake in 350°F oven about 35 minutes or until top springs back when lightly touched.
   This can also be made in small tart pans, baking for about 15 to 20 minutes.

Rum Cup Custard

Save this recipe for special occasions and holidays.

Serves Two

1 cup low-fat milk
¼ cup nonfat dry powdered milk
    pinch of salt
½ teaspoon vanilla extract
½ teaspoon rum extract

1 egg
1½ teaspoons honey
    dash of cinnamon
    dash of nutmeg

1. Combine milks, salt, vanilla, and rum extract.
2. In a separate bowl, blend egg and honey. Slowly add milk mixture and blend well.
3. Pour mixture into 2 custard cups. Sprinkle each with cinnamon and nutmeg.
4. Place custard cups in pan with 1 inch of hot water.
5. Bake about 50 minutes in 325°F oven until knife inserted in center comes out clean.

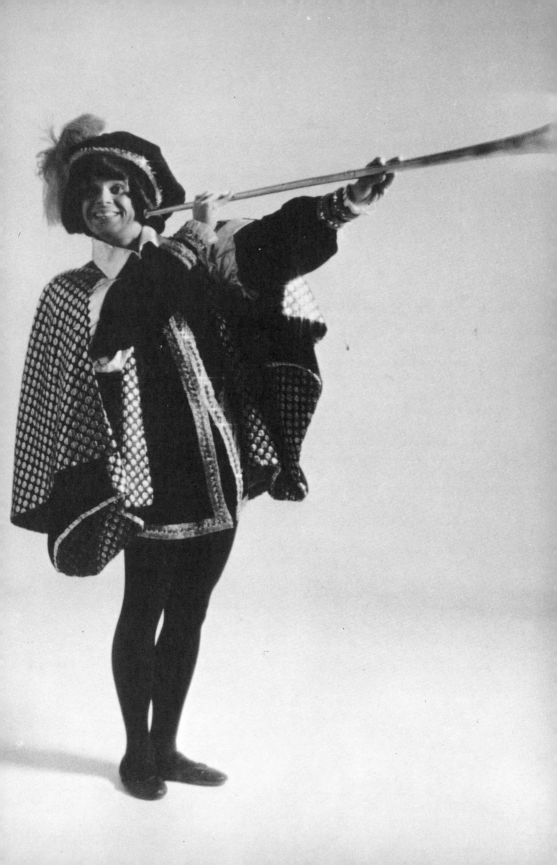

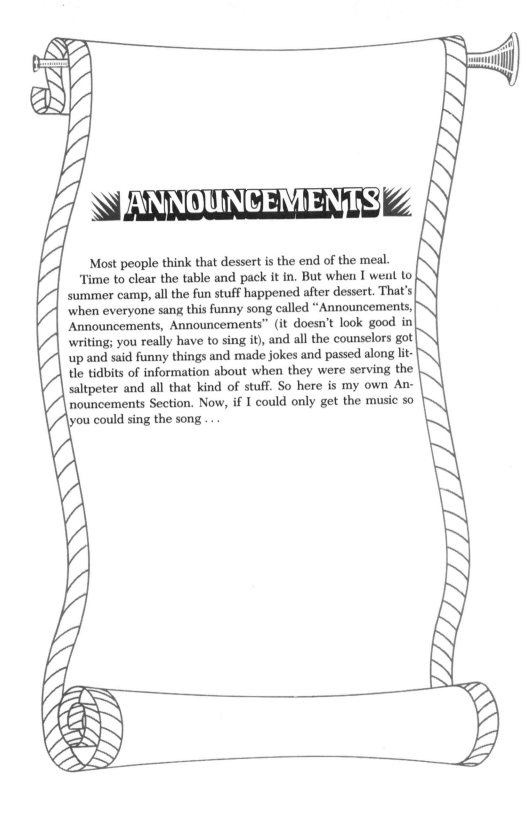

ANNOUNCEMENTS

Most people think that dessert is the end of the meal.
Time to clear the table and pack it in. But when I went to summer camp, all the fun stuff happened after dessert. That's when everyone sang this funny song called "Announcements, Announcements, Announcements" (it doesn't look good in writing; you really have to sing it), and all the counselors got up and said funny things and made jokes and passed along little tidbits of information about when they were serving the saltpeter and all that kind of stuff. So here is my own Announcements Section. Now, if I could only get the music so you could sing the song . . .

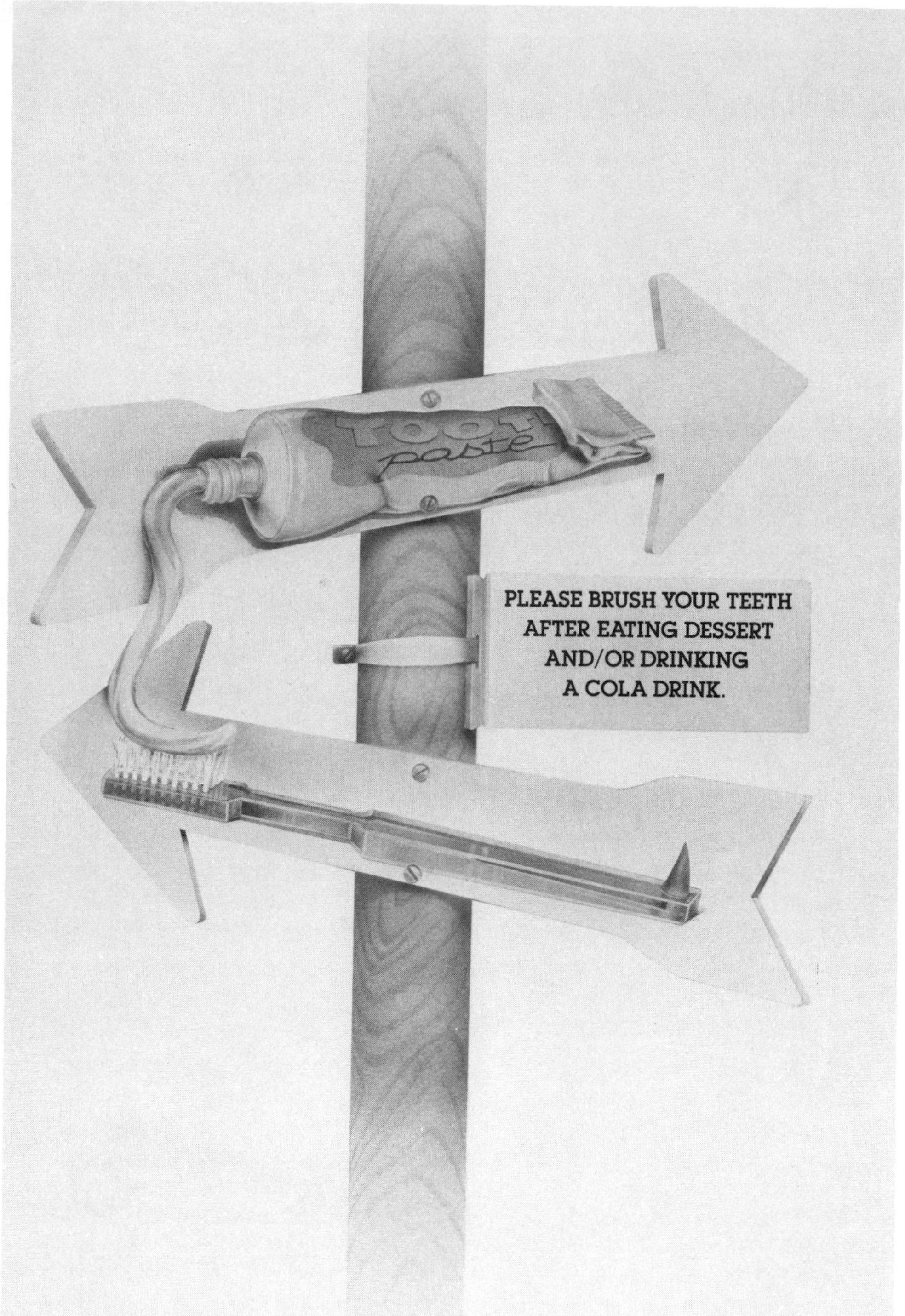

PLEASE BRUSH YOUR TEETH
AFTER EATING DESSERT
AND/OR DRINKING
A COLA DRINK.

Your family weekend morning weigh-in chart for two weeks:

Member of family	Sat.	Sun.	Sat.	Sun.
(Your name here)	(Your weight)		(Your weight)	

date here _____ _____ _____ _____

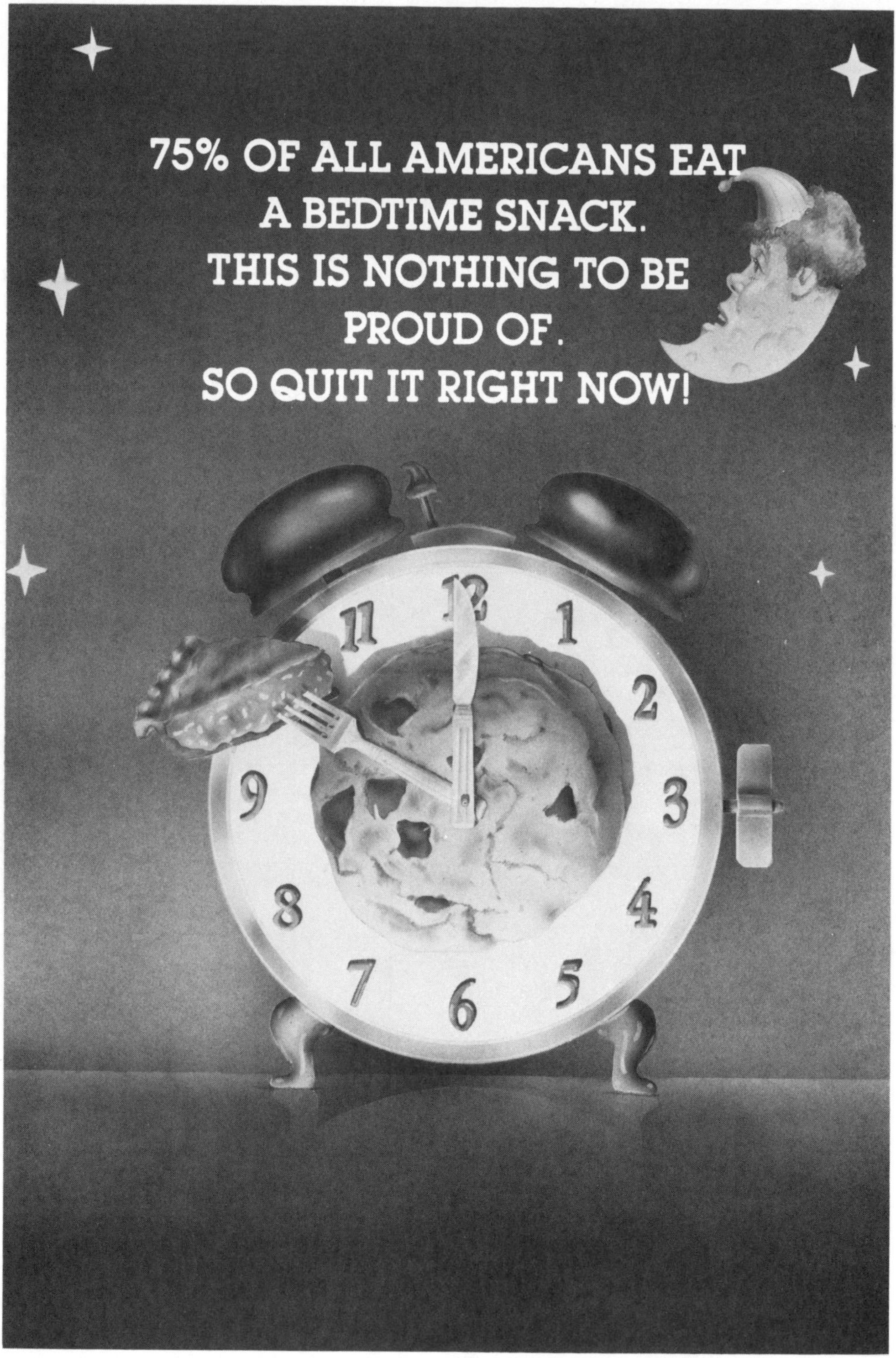
75% OF ALL AMERICANS EAT
A BEDTIME SNACK.
THIS IS NOTHING TO BE
PROUD OF.
SO QUIT IT RIGHT NOW!

PUT DOWN THAT CUP OF COFFEE!

PORTIONS FOR LOSERS

We all know that the Live-It is a volume food plan, so that the amount of what you eat matters even more than the content of said food. So how much is the right amount? I can only give you some basic outlines. After all, I don't believe you should walk around with a calorie counter in your handbag, a computer up your sleeve, and a digital calculator with a separate scale to figure these things out. I've just got a few rules that I go by that are more common sense than anything else.

- If you leave the table feeling stuffed, you probably ate too much.
- If the recipe is for six people and you eat half of it by yourself—guess what? You ate too much.
- The right portion when you're eating a breast of chicken is one breast of chicken—skin off, please.
- The right portion for a container of yogurt is one container of yogurt.
- Man cannot live by cottage cheese alone, so ½ cup will do.
- If you're eating a potato, eat one medium potato.
- If you're eating bread, one slice will do nicely, thank you.
- Basta on the pasta—only ½ cup and not too often.
- If you're using butter, one pat, please.
- If you're eating red meat, two slices should do nicely. Or one, if it's larger, but it should be under 4 ounces, cooked.
- Dressing on the side, please: Just wet the dry areas—don't keep wetting the wet areas.
- If you splurge on a cookie, have one cookie. Not a bag of cookies.
- Fish shrinks up when you cook it, and since it's sold by weight anyway, you should ask for 6 to 8 ounces of fish fillets. (4 ounces after cooking.)

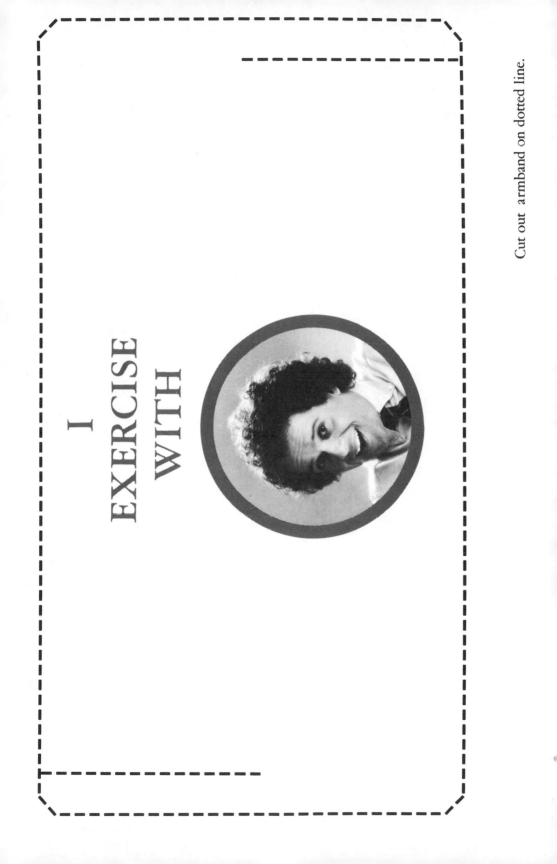

I
EXERCISE
WITH

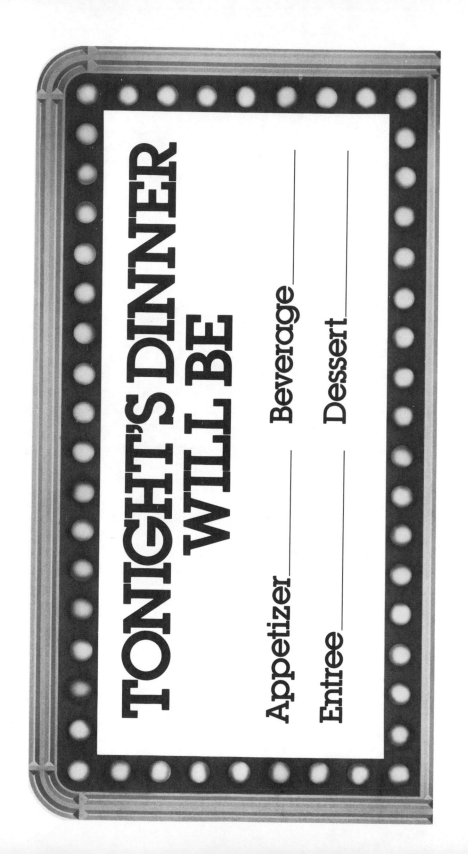

Index

red, 17–18, 76, 132, 204
  See also Beef; Lamb; Pork
Melamud, Judy, 146
Melon. *See* Cantaloupe, fresh fruit cups
Menu planning, 132–35
Meringue pie, lemoniest, 194–95
Microwave ovens, 175
Midmorning break. *See* Breaks
Milk, 20
  banana smoothie, 47
  -based soups, 177, 179
  bread pudding, 192
  Caribbean cocktail, 50
  cheeseless cheesecake, 193
  fruity shake, 91
  quickie quiche, 83
  rum cup custard, 197
Mind, Live-It, 25
Mineral water, 76
Minestrone soup, 177
Mixmaster, 24
Mock sour cream, 161
  rolled sole amandine, 151
Mold, chilly cottage cheese, 87
Monosodium glutamate, 135
Monterrey Jack cheese. *See* Jack cheese
Morning, 27–51
  the blues, 28
  Breakfast Pledge, 27
  Breakfast Quiz, 29–31
  clean up and clear up checklist, 41–42
  profiles, 28, 30–31
  schedules for, 40–41
    exercise and stretch, 31–39
Mozzarella cheese:
  chicken, 141
  yummy breakfast quiche, 51
MSG, 135
Muenster cheese, spinach roll-ups, 150
Muffins, eggs McSimmons, 46
Mushrooms:
  chicken sesame, 144
  fresh, salad, 167
  overnight salad, 165
  rolled sole amandine, 151
  Search for Tomato, 100
  storage of, 18–19
  stuffed, 99
  vegetable salad, 171
  warm cabbage salad, 170–71
  yummy breakfast quiche, 51
Mustard, 21
  dressing, 161

Neck exercises, 117–22
  chew-man-chew, 118
  pout-ers, 117
  vowel stretchers, 119–20
  wrinkle wipes, 120–21
Neufchâtel cheese, 21
  apple-blossom sandwich, 91
  General Hospitality Rx, 103
  zany zucchini, 99
Never-Say-Diet (Simmons), 11, 12, 14, 16
Never-Say-Diet Cookbook (Simmons), 11–12
  sources of recipes in, 12–14
Niçoise salad, 156
No-kidding ketchup, 161
Not-so-chilly chili, 93
Nuñez, Anita Rena, 194

Oils:
  cooking, 20
  for salad dressing, 160
  See also Salad(s); Salad dressings
Olives:
  General Hospitality Rx, 103
  overnight Salad, 165
  tuna salad, special, 165
Omelets:
  ricotta, 46
  strawberry, 43
One Loaf to Live, 101
Onion(s):
  soup, 177
  storage of, 19
  stuffed mushrooms, 99
  yummy breakfast quiche, 51
Orange(s):
  chicken, 142–43
  fresh fruit cups, 47
  fruited curry luncheon salad, 81
  vinaigrette, 162
  wild watercress salad, 167
Orange juice, 76
  orange chicken, 142–43
  orange cream puffs, 191
  vinaigrette, 162
Organ meats, 18
Overnight salad, 165

Pancakes, perfect, 51
Parsley:
  storage of, 19
  tabouleh-stuffed cucumbers, 85
Parties, 137–38
Pasta, 19

Young and the Ratatouille, 98
yummy breakfast quiche, 51
Tootsie rolls, 64
Tossed salad, 156
Tryptophan, 177
Tuna:
  imperial, 86
  packed in oil,.19
  salad, special, 165
Tupperware, 89
Turkey, 17
  Chinese, salad, 169
  eggs McSimmons, 46
  fruited curry luncheon salad, 81
  One Loaf to Live, 101
  ricotta omelet, 146
  soup, 177
Turnovers:
  apple, filo-dough, 102–103
  As the World, 102

Vegetable oils, 20, 160
Vegetables, 20, 132, 135
  creamy cauliflower, 151
  salad, 171
  storage of, 18–19
  stuffed bell peppers, 86
  stuffed zucchini, 84–85
  See also Salad(s)
V-8 juice, chicken zucchini soup, 181
Vichyssoise, 177
Vinegar:
  fresh mushroom salad dressing, 167
  no-kidding ketchup, 161
  orange vinaigrette, 162
  overnight salad, marinade for, 165
  poppy seed dressing, 162
  Roquefort dressing, 162
  spicy, dressing, 131
  tarragon dressing, 163
Vowel stretchers, 119–20

Waldorf salad, 156
Walnut oil, 20
Warm cabbage salad, 170–71
Warm-ups, 58, 67
Warne, Karen, 84
Water, 131

Water chestnuts:
  Chinese chicken salad, 169
  seven-layer salad, 166–67
Watercress, wild, salad, 167
Weather and your skin, 122
Weekend lunches, 108–109
Weigh-in chart, 202
Wild watercress salad, 167
Wind, 122
Wine, 109, 130
Wok, 22, 135
Wonton soup, 177
Worry, 122
Wrinkle wipes, 120–21
Wrinkles, 122

Yogurt, 20
  apple apricot dream soup, 180–81
  frozen, 189
    fruit salad (popsticks), 192
  General Hospitality Rx, 103
  grapefruit cups, 49
  hurry-up fruit shake, 50–51
  portion size, 204
  salad dressings:
    for Chinese chicken salad, 169
    cucumber-and-, delight, 164
    fruit salad topping, 160
    mock sour cream, 161
    Roquefort, 162
  strawberry egg cakes, 49
  tomato salad, 173
Young and the Ratatouille, 98
Yummy breakfast quiche, 51

Zucchini:
  carrot cake, 196–97
  chicken soup, 181
  macho gazpacho, 178
  quickie quiche, 83
  Search for Tomato, 100
  stuffed, 84–85
  stuffed mushrooms, 99
  vegetable salad, 171
  warm cabbage salad, 170–71
  the Young and the Ratatouille, 98
  zany, 99
Zuniga, Betty, 92